Sarah Ockwell-Smith is the mother of four children. She has a BSc in Psychology and worked for several years in pharmaceutical research and development. Following the birth of her first child, Sarah re-trained as an antenatal teacher and birth and postnatal doula. She has also undertaken training in hypnotherapy and psychotherapy. Sarah specialises in gentle parenting methods and is co-founder of the Gentle Parenting website www.gentleparenting.co.uk. She also blogs at www.sarahockwell-smith.com.

Sarah is the author of twelve other parenting books: *Baby-Calm, ToddlerCalm, The Gentle Sleep Book, The Gentle Parenting Book, Why Your Baby's Sleep Matters, The Gentle Discipline Book, The Gentle Potty Training Book, The Gentle Eating Book, The Second Baby Book, The Starting School Book, Between* and *How to Be a Calm Parent*. She frequently writes for magazines and newspapers, and is often called upon as a parenting expert for national television and radio.

SARAH OCKWELL-SMITH

BEGINNINGS

A guide to
child psychology and development
for parents of 0–5-year-olds

PIATKUS

PIATKUS

First published in Great Britain in 2022 by Piatkus

1 3 5 7 9 10 8 6 4 2

A CIP catalogue record for this book
is available from the British Library.

ISBN 978-0-349-43128-4

Illustrations by Andrassy Media
Designed and typeset by EM&EN
Printed and bound in Great Britain by Clays Ltd, Elcograf S.p.A

Papers used by Piatkus are from well-managed forests
and other responsible sources.

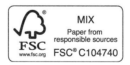

PIATKUS
An imprint of
Little, Brown Book Group
Carmelite House
50 Victoria Embankment
London EC4Y 0DZ

An Hachette UK Company
www.hachette.co.uk

Contents

Introduction

The first five years of a child's life underpin their future personality, health and relationships. In that time – just under two thousand days – a child's body and brain will grow and change far quicker than at any other time in their life. The way that parents and carers respond to them during these years has more of an impact on their development than anything else. We are the architects of their lives. An exciting yet terrifying thought, isn't it?

Surprisingly, many parents and carers are unaware of what is happening in their child's brain and how they are developing, perhaps because the relevant information is so often written in dull medical jargon, or only found in weighty textbooks. Over the last two decades, I have been asked thousands of times if I can recommend a book about child development – one that covers the common queries about physical development, such as, 'How does a baby learn to walk?' as well as, 'How do children learn to talk?' and questions about brain development. Parents and carers want to understand what neurological stages their children are going through and how this affects their behaviour. They want to be better informed so they can help their children to blossom into confident and happy individuals who will meet their full potential. But they just don't have the time to trawl through a three-hundred-page textbook to do so. And rightly so – they have other things to do!

Beginnings was born out of a desire to fill this gap and provide parents and carers with the information that they're desperate for, in a way that is not too technical, but not patronising either. It's the book I wish I had read when my own four children were small – and the one I hope *they* will read in the future, when they have children of their own.

So what will you find in this book? We start with a chapter on life in utero, providing descriptions of how a foetus develops and grows, with an emphasis on the astounding brain development that occurs during this period. Chapters 2 to 5 divide the first year of life up into blocks of three months. There are so many incredible changes in the first year that to do justice to them, we need to break the chapters down into smaller age periods. Chapters 6 and 7 look at life from the first to the second birthday, as babyhood comes to an end and the beginnings of toddlerhood emerge. Chapter 8 considers the fascinating world of two-year-olds, while Chapter 9 deals with the development that takes place once a child turns three. Finally, Chapter 10 is a study of four-year-olds, right up to their fifth birthdays.

As you move through this book, you will notice that each chapter is broken down into the following:

- Brain development – changes that take place in the brain and neurological growth

- Physical development – what happens to your child's body, including physical milestones

- Feeding and eating development – your child's relationship with food at the various stages and physical changes in their body that affect eating

- Sleep development – how sleep varies at different ages, including sleep milestones and how these are affected by physical, neurological and psychological development

- Social and psychological development – how your child experiences and interacts with the world around them, and their relationships with yourself and others close to them

- Language development – how your child learns to communicate, including the emergence of talking and elements that influence it

- Play ideas – to help your child to develop, bond with you and, most importantly, keep them entertained.

These sections will make it easier for you to skip straight to any areas of special interest or find answers to any pressing questions you may have when you don't have time to read the whole chapter.

As well as longer descriptions of physiological and psychological development, you will also find the following throughout the book:

- **Neuroscience Nuggets** – small, easily digestible, bites of brain science

- **Fun Facts** – interesting and entertaining facts and figures

- **Anthropology Titbits** – beliefs and behaviours concerning childhood from different cultures around the world and from different periods of history

- **Parenting Q&As** – common questions that parents ask me (and my answers)

- **Parent Observations** – real-life experience from other parents

- **Quotes** – child-development-related quotes from well-known figures, past and present

Finally, at the end of the book you will find some suggested further reading, if you would like to expand your knowledge.

Important note on using this book

Milestones are unique to each child. Throughout this book I refer to averages in development; however, it is important to understand that some children will hit these milestones earlier and some later.

If your child was born prematurely, then (at least for the earlier chapters) please go by their due date, not their birth date, when considering milestones.

Also, the statistics in this book refer to children who are neurotypical (i.e. follow a pattern of typical neurological development), and while many of the descriptions in the book will still apply to children who are neurodivergent (those who differ from the typical patterns due to autism, attention deficit disorder or similar), please keep in mind that your child is not a number, and they shouldn't be judged against them either. All children are different, and it is important to focus on your own child's unique curve.

If you are concerned about your child hitting their milestones, please speak to a professional, such as your family doctor, paediatrician, midwife or health visitor. This book is not intended as a substitute for professional psychological or medical advice.

1
Life in Utero

There is arguably nothing quite so astounding as the beginnings of a new life. In a mere 280 days (or thereabouts), an embryo containing just one cell grows to a newborn containing twenty-six billion cells! But life in utero isn't just about growing physically. Plenty of psychological development happens, too, including the start of the important attachment that will link you and your child together for a lifetime of love.

A quick note on terminology

Four different terms recur throughout this chapter: embryo, foetus, newborn and baby. The word embryo is used to describe the very earliest stages, from a single cell through to Week 11 of pregnancy (which is actually week nine of development, since a pregnancy is dated from the first day of the last menstrual period, usually two weeks before conception). From Week 11, the embryo becomes a foetus, and once the foetus is born, he or she then becomes a newborn (or neonate). Use of the word baby is more about personal choice, based upon beliefs, rather than medical terminology; some will choose to use it from conception, some wait until the foetal stage, while others wait until birth.

In this chapter, we will look at the brain – how it grows and begins to form the connections that lead to learning and the forming of personality. We will consider physical development, too, and how an embryo goes from a tiny tadpole-shaped tube to a pumpkin-sized newborn. Finally, we will reflect on how you can bond with – and play with – your baby before they are even born.

How the brain develops in utero

Only three weeks after conception, the building blocks of the brain (known as the neural tube) start to develop, via a process known as neurulation. The neural tube, which looks a little like a tadpole (you can see an illustration below), forms the very beginnings of the embryo's brain and spinal cord. Only a week or two later, the neural tube will close and become the distinct parts, which are the brain, skull, spine and spinal cord.

The brain grows from stem cells, which develop into the two main cell types of the brain, known as neurons and glia.

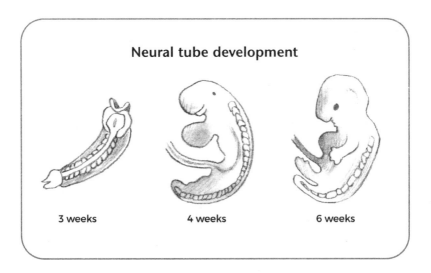

Neural tube development

3 weeks   4 weeks   6 weeks

Neuroscience Nugget The first electrical activity in the embryo's brain occurs only six weeks after conception.

Neurons function as the communication centre of the brain, passing messages from one area to another, while glia provide chemical and structural support to aid this process. New neuron development is known as neurogenesis, while new glia development is known as gliogenesis. Neurogenesis is ongoing throughout our lives, but the most neurons are undoubtedly formed during infancy.

Brain development in the first trimester (Weeks 1–11)

During the first trimester (months one to three) of pregnancy, the brain is focused on growing and multiplying the number of neurons. When the neural tube closes, around the sixth week of pregnancy, the rounded section at the top starts to form the three distinct parts of the brain: the forebrain, the midbrain and the hindbrain. While the whole of the brain increases rapidly in size during this period, the forebrain is by far the largest section.

By the end of the first trimester, the brain and skull are more recognisably round and the main three areas further develop into the cerebrum (the largest part of the brain, controlling voluntary muscle movement, emotions, speech and

Neuroscience Nugget When a baby is born, their brain contains around one hundred billion neurons. That's about the same as the total number of stars in our Milky Way.

thinking), the cerebellum (a smaller section, responsible for movement, co-ordination and balance), the hypothalamus (which controls body temperature) and the pituitary gland (a tiny pea-sized area of the brain, responsible for growth and the control of hormones).

Brain development in the second trimester (Weeks 12–23)

In the second trimester, neurons begin to move around the brain in a process known as migration. This allows them to travel to their final position in the brain, ready to perform their communication duties there. Towards the end of the second trimester, the neurons start to form branches, called

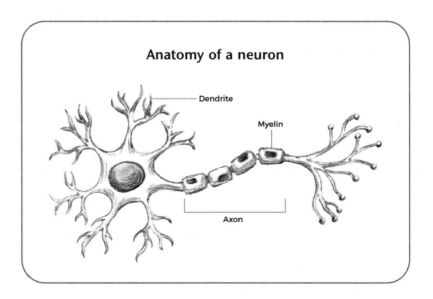

Anatomy of a neuron

Dendrite

Myelin

Axon

dendrites, and a long cable-like structure, called an axon. These dendrites and axons allow the neurons to send and receive messages through a system of chemical and electrical impulses. A further process, called myelination, covers the axons in a fatty substance known as a myelin sheath, which acts as a form of insulation, helping the electrical signals in the axons to travel more quickly.

This combination of neural development and the separation of the brain into distinct parts (particularly the cerebellum) allows the foetus to take control of their bodily movements, with purposeful stretching and kicking. Between the fourth and fifth months into the pregnancy, the foetus starts to suck and swallow and practise breathing movements, as a result of their brain directing their diaphragm and chest muscles to contract.

By the end of the second trimester, the basic structure of the foetus's brain is similar to that of an adult, although there is still a way to go.

Brain development in the third trimester (Weeks 24–40)

In the final trimester of pregnancy, the foetal brain grows rapidly, starting at around 85g at month six and ending up around 400g at birth – around a tenth of the newborn's body weight. During this period, it also separates into two sides,

FUN FACT
fMRI (functional magnetic resonance imaging) is a relatively new imaging technology that allows scientists to study the connections in the growing brain before the baby is even born.[1]

Neuroscience Nugget In utero, a foetus's brain grows 250,000 nerve cells per minute.[2]

known as hemispheres. Maturation of all areas of the brain continues, and by the thirty-second week of pregnancy, the foetus's hypothalamus is mature enough to independently control their body temperature and breathing.

In the third trimester, more mature neurons start to produce chemicals known as neurotransmitters, which will

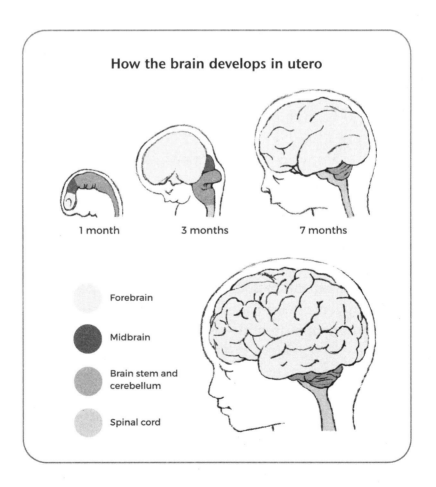

How the brain develops in utero

1 month   3 months   7 months

Forebrain

Midbrain

Brain stem and cerebellum

Spinal cord

ultimately allow communication between the neurons to occur; however, while the foetus is still in utero, the neuro-transmitters focus on growth, rather than communication. Initially, they send messages to the neurons to connect with each other by building plug-like structures known as synapses. This concentration on what's known as synaptic connection puts the structure in place for more sophisticated communication once the baby is born.

Until the start of the third trimester, the brain is relatively smooth in appearance. It's only at the end of pregnancy that the characteristic walnut-like folds fully form in the cerebrum. These folds and indentations – called sulci, and known collectively as the cerebral cortex – give the cerebrum a much greater surface area, without taking up more space in the skull. You can clearly see the changes in the foetal brain, including the development of sulci, in the diagram opposite.

Physical development in utero

While your baby's brain is busy growing, the rest of their body is undergoing tremendous change, too. At the very beginning of pregnancy, an embryo is as tiny as a poppy seed, growing over the next nine months to the size of a pumpkin. The embryo's cells receive instructions from the molecules they contain, and also signals from other cells, which tell them what they should grow into – anything from an intestine to a fingernail.

A new baby is like the beginning of all things
– wonder, hope, a dream of possibilities.
Eda LaShan, American writer

> **FUN FACT**
> *An embryo's heart starts to beat around the fifth to sixth week of pregnancy, and by the ninth week, it beats at between 140 and 170 beats per minute, double the average adult heart rate.*

Let's take a look at the main physical development that occurs over the three trimesters of pregnancy.

Physical development in the first trimester

By the fifth week of pregnancy, the embryo is comprised of three layers, known as the ectoderm, mesoderm and endoderm. The endoderm is the innermost layer and will eventually become the intestines and lungs; the mesoderm – the middle layer – will become the heart and circulatory system, the kidneys, bones and reproductive organs; and the ectoderm will become the skin, eyes, ears and central nervous system.

By Week 7, the embryo has small arm and leg buds, a more recognisable head shape and the beginnings of eyes, ears, a nose and a mouth. By Week 9, fingers and toes are forming, although they are joined by webbing, along with elbows, as

> **FUN FACT**
> *Although all babies are born with twenty teeth, these do not usually make their way through the gums until several months after birth. However, around one in 2,000 to 3,000 babies are born with 'natal teeth' that have already come through.*

the arm and leg buds become much more arm- and leg-like. By Week 12, the head has taken on a characteristic round shape and is approximately half of the total length of the now foetus. Eyelids are discernible, although they are fused closed for now. Fingernails begin to sprout and the webbing on the fingers and toes starts to disappear. Tooth buds start to form in the mouth by Week 10, and finally, by Week 11, the beginnings of external genitalia are in evidence.

Physical development in the second trimester

As a foetus enters into the second trimester, they are recognisable as a baby, although they are still very skinny as they have yet to lay down fat stores; these will start to accumulate as they progress through the second trimester.

Towards the end of the second trimester, the foetus's lungs begin to form air sacs known as alveoli, although their lungs are still immature and will develop further in the third trimester. Eyebrows, eyelashes and hair on the head start to grow at

---

PARENTING Q&A

Q. *I am twenty weeks pregnant but haven't felt my baby kick yet. Why is this?*

A. *Most people will feel their baby kick at some point between Weeks 16 and 24. However, first-time mums tend to feel kicks later. When you feel kicks also depends on the position your baby is lying in and where your placenta is located. If it is at the front of your uterus (known as an anterior placenta), this can disguise the baby's kicks.*

this stage, and towards the end of the second trimester, fine hair – known as lanugo – will grow all over their body. The lanugo acts to protect the foetus's skin while they are in utero and has usually mostly disappeared by the time of the birth. Any remaining lanugo at that stage will quickly fall out.

Vernix caseosa, commonly known just as vernix – a greasy white substance, made from skin cells and excretions from sebaceous glands – starts to develop around the twentieth week and continues to build throughout the second trimester. Vernix protects the foetus's skin and helps to waterproof it, and the lanugo (the fine hair on the foetus's body) helps it to stick.

Physical development in the third trimester

During the third trimester the foetus's body fat builds up dramatically, increasing their weight fivefold during this period. Their lungs mature further, as more alveoli form and a substance known as surfactant, made from protein and fats, is secreted, helping the air sacs to stay inflated. During pregnancy, the foetus's lungs are filled with fluid, which will be released when they are born, helped by the process of crying. Until the moment of birth, they receive all the oxygen they need from the mother's blood.

By Week 28, the foetus's eyelids are no longer fused, and they will open their eyes for the first time. Although there is little to see in the uterus, they can sense changes in light through the uterine wall.

Most babies will turn head down and start to engage into the mother's pelvis by Week 36, as gravity pulls the heaviest part of the body – the skull – downwards. The bones in the skull are still soft and unfused; the fibrous connections between them are known as cranial sutures and the two diamond-shaped

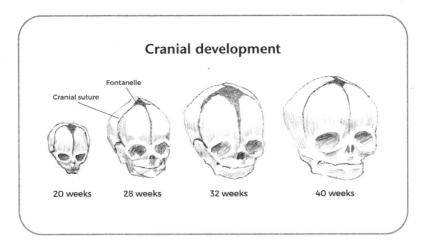

Cranial development

Fontanelle

Cranial suture

20 weeks   28 weeks   32 weeks   40 weeks

holes – one at the front of the skull (known as anterior) and one at the back (posterior) – are called fontanelles. This flexibility allows the skull plates to overlap each other, to make the skull smaller for an easier birth, as well as enabling the skull to continue growing throughout childhood. We will talk a little more about fontanelles in the next chapter.

Vernix continues to build until around Week 34, when it starts to break down in the amniotic fluid and the foetus then swallows and excretes it, so there is little left by the end of the pregnancy. Despite this, babies are usually born with a thin coating of vernix, although the further after their due date they arrive, the less vernix there will be.

FUN FACT
Vernix is a great natural moisturiser that can also help to protect the baby's skin from bacterial infections, which is why the World Health Organization recommends not wiping it off or washing a newborn in the first twenty-four hours.

How big is your baby?[3]

Week	Average weight	Average length	Equivalent to
4	–	–	Poppy seed
8	1g	1.6cm	Raspberry
12	14g	5.4cm	Lime
16	100g	11.6cm	Avocado
20	343g	25.6cm	Pomegranate
24	662g	30.6cm	Cantaloupe melon
28	1.1kg	37.6cm	Aubergine
32	1.9kg	42.4cm	Pineapple
36	2.6kg	49.8cm	Honeydew melon
40	3.5kg	51.2cm	Pumpkin

What causes labour to start?

While most babies are born within two to three weeks of their estimated due date, fewer than 5 per cent arrive on that date. Scientists aren't entirely sure what causes labour to start, but research suggests that it is likely due to the levels of surfactant released by the foetus's lungs, indicating that they are ready to be born.[4] Further research has found that the amniotic fluid contains more telomeres (a part of DNA involved in ageing) as the due date approaches, indicating that it is time for the pregnancy to end, so it seems likely that it is a combination of factors, both foetal and maternal, that ultimately decide when labour will happen.[5]

Feeding and eating in utero

For the first week after conception, the embryo receives all its nutrients from the endometrium (the lining of the uterus), which remains a significant source of nutrition for most of the first trimester, while the placenta is developing. During the second and third trimesters, the foetus gets all the nourishment they need from the placenta.

Although a foetus does not actively eat during pregnancy, they still learn to drink, by swallowing amniotic fluid (fluid

---

The amazing placenta

The placenta provides the foetus with oxygen and all the necessary nutrients, such as glucose and vitamins. It also removes waste products, such as carbon dioxide, and produces hormones to help the foetus grow. The placenta also protects the foetus from any infections in the mother and enables antibodies to pass through from the maternal bloodstream.

When conception occurs, the blastocyst (the developmental stage from conception to two weeks, before an embryo forms) embeds into the uterine wall and the placenta is formed from this combination of the blastocyst and uterine tissue. One side of the placenta is fixed to the wall of the uterus, while the other is joined to the foetus via the umbilical cord. The placenta's formation is complete by the twentieth week of pregnancy, but it continues to grow throughout the remaining weeks. At birth, most placentas weigh around 700g and are around the size of a frisbee.

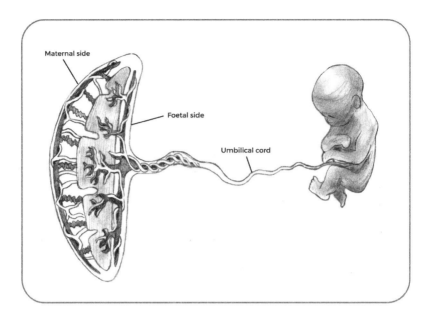

in the uterus which helps to protect the foetus as they grow). Until the middle of the second trimester, amniotic fluid is composed of water from the mother, after twenty weeks, however, the fluid is composed entirely of foetal urine produced when the foetus swallows and excretes it. In fact, by the end of pregnancy, the entire amount of amniotic fluid is recycled by the foetus (through a process of swallowing and peeing) every three hours. Amniotic fluid is at its greatest level by around Week 34 of pregnancy, when it averages around 800ml, dropping to around 600ml at birth.

FUN FACT
The taste of amniotic fluid depends on what the mother eats, with things like garlic changing it, and also making acceptance of that flavour more likely once the baby is born and starts to eat solid foods, according to research.[6]

By Week 16 of pregnancy, taste buds are fully developed and the foetus is able to taste the amniotic fluid and differentiate different flavours within it.

PARENTING Q&A

Q. *I have read that some mothers eat the placenta once their baby is born, and this is said to help their recovery. Is there any evidence for this?*

A. *Placentophagy (eating the placenta) is common in many mammals, although rare in humans. Over the last few years, however, it has become more popular, with many mothers claiming it helped them to recover their energy and balance their postnatal hormones.[7] The two main ways people consume their placentas are by blending small chunks of it raw in a smoothie or by dehydrating and grinding it, consuming the powder via capsules. As there are some concerns about the hygiene risks involved, many parents prefer to employ the services of a professional placenta encapsulation specialist, rather than make the smoothies or capsules themselves, although this can be quite expensive.*

FUN FACT

Some parents choose not to cut the umbilical cord once the baby is born, leaving it attached to the placenta (which is covered in herbs, to give it a scent, wrapped in a cloth and carried with the baby) until the cord naturally falls off within a few days. This process, known as 'lotus birth', is believed to be a gentler transition for the baby.

FUN FACT
Life in utero is pretty noisy, what with the maternal heartbeat and digestive sounds and muffled voices. Newborns often sleep better when these sorts of noises are played around them, rather than putting them down to sleep in a silent room.

Sleep development in utero

Understandably, it is quite tricky to research foetal sleep, as it is impossible to measure foetal brain activity directly while they are in utero. But scientists believe that it mimics adult sleep as the pregnancy progresses. Research studying foetal heart rates suggests that sleep patterns are well established by the thirtieth week of pregnancy.[8] Further research suggests that rapid eye movement sleep (REM) starts around the seventh month of pregnancy.[9] REM sleep is important for brain development, particularly neural connections, and to enable the foetus to process the environment in which they live.

Foetuses spend most of their time in utero asleep – between 85 and 95 per cent of the time in the third trimester, which is similar to the amount they will sleep as newborns.

Social and psychological development in utero

When do personality and consciousness form? Does a sense of self and awareness start in the newborn period? Later? Or perhaps earlier, while the foetus is still in the womb? These are questions that have puzzled psychologists and philosophers the world over and naturally, they are tricky to answer.

Parent Observation 'When I was pregnant my baby was always very active just after lunch every day; now she is here, she has the same wide-awake period every day, at exactly the same time she went crazy during my pregnancy.'

What we do know, is that when the brain has matured to a certain point, with communication between both hemispheres and significant neural connections in place, then, arguably, there is a chance that consciousness may develop. This is most likely at some point during the third trimester, when the neurological building blocks, although rudimentary, are in place.

Some prenatal psychologists (those interested in pre-birth development) believe that personality does indeed start in the womb and that the shared experiences of mother and child during pregnancy influence future personality. Research has found that the levels of maternal stress in pregnancy, for instance, can potentially result in more advanced neurological development in the baby once born.[10] This doesn't mean that lots of stress is great for foetuses – far from it – but it does indicate that a foetus is affected by life before birth, with what can be a lasting impact on their brain and, as further research has shown, their temperament as a newborn.[11]

Everything grows rounder and wider and weirder,
and I sit here in the middle of it all and wonder
who in the world you will turn out to be.
Carrie Fisher, American actress

Neuroscience Nugget Playing music to your bump has several lasting effects on their brain, from helping them to be calmer once they are born to increasing the chance of them being musical as they grow.[12] Research has found that the two pieces of music that foetuses respond to the most are Mozart's 'Eine kleine Nachtmusik' and Queen's 'Bohemian Rhapsody'.[13]

Language development in utero

While language doesn't truly start until a baby is born, they are still learning in utero. A foetus can hear their parents and others speaking – their mother's voice becomes incredibly familiar to them because the sound of her speaking is amplified into the uterus. Foetuses respond to the musical aspects of speech, and a mother may notice that they are more active while they are speaking or singing. This pre-birth language experience provides a solid foundation for the development of communication after birth.

FUN FACT
Accents may develop in utero. Research has found that the cries of newborns with French parents are different to those of newborns whose parents are German, indicating that the foetus may already be noticing the patterns of their parents' voices while in utero.[14]

Play ideas during pregnancy

It's never too early to play with your baby. Prenatal play is focused on bonding and building an attachment. You probably 'play' with them already without realising, with unconscious actions such as:

- rubbing your bump when your baby kicks
- talking to your bump
- singing to your bump
- playing a piece of your favourite music for your bump while you lie down, relax and close your eyes, focusing on your breathing
- visualising your baby, now and once they are born.

These everyday activities will help to kickstart the bond with your baby once they are born.

Soon, the foetus's dark, aquatic world, in which they are kept at a constant temperature, have never experienced hunger or thirst and where they are constantly in physical contact with

Anthropology Titbit In Mexico, some mothers wear a bola necklace (also known as *'llamador de angeles'* or an 'angel caller'). Thought to originate in Indonesia, it is a long silver chain with a chime ball at the end, which sits on the bump, gently chiming for the baby as the mother moves around. This ancient Mayan custom is said to calm both the unborn baby and its mother.

Parent Observation 'I used to listen to a birthing relaxation track every evening during my pregnancy. I think my son must remember the music because it always calms him down and helps him to sleep when I play it now.'

PARENTING Q&A

Q. *My partner is bonding well with her bump, but I don't feel a connection with the baby yet. Is there anything I can do to help?*

A. *First of all, don't worry if you don't feel a connection with your baby yet; this is quite common before birth. It's hard to bond with somebody you have never met, so please don't beat yourself up. One thing you could do that might help is to read a bedtime story to your baby every night. It doesn't have to be long – just a page or two – but research has shown that foetuses do recognise their parents' voices, and this could really help you bond when the baby is born, if not before.*[15]

another human will come to an end. The only world they have ever known will shortly be replaced by a brand-new life in air – full of bright lights, changing temperatures and new sensations – and one where, ultimately, they will have to learn how to be alone. The transition from womb to world is the biggest we will ever make in our lives. Chapter 2 explores these changes and challenges and will help you to understand life for your newborn and how to make the transition as calm and as easy as possible.

2

Birth to Three Months

Your baby is finally here. Congratulations!

Nothing is quite like the feeling of holding that warm little bundle in your arms for the first time, trying to work out who they look like, what name suits them most, what their personality is like and who they will grow to be. There is such opportunity ahead and a whole world of possibilities for your son or daughter.

The first three months are all about getting to know each other, and your baby transitioning to life outside the womb. Many refer to this time as 'the fourth trimester', a term used to describe the early weeks when the newborn is still very foetus-like (you will notice they still curl up as if they are inside the uterus) and getting used to the world after birth. Later in this chapter, we will consider some ways to use the idea of the fourth trimester to help your baby to be calmer; let's start, however, with a look at how babies experience birth.

The moment of birth

When we speak about birth experiences in our society, all attention is focused on the parents. But the baby also goes through birth. What is it like for them? That's a question that we will never fully be able to answer, but we know that they will encounter a great deal of pressure and squeezing all over

Anthropology Titbit In the Netherlands, new parents welcome the arrival of a baby by eating a snack known as *beschuit met muisjes* (biscuits with mice) – small rusk-type biscuits covered with the traditional *muisjes* (mice) bread topping, comprising tiny balls of liquorice, similar to hundreds and thousands. Male babies are welcomed with blue and white *muisjes*, and female babies are welcomed with pink and white ones.

their body, which helps to prepare their lungs to expel any fluid and to take their first breath of air when they are born. Later in this chapter, we will speak about the dramatic differences between the baby's 'womb world' and life outside the uterus, and how understanding this enormous transition can help parents and carers to calm and soothe them, but there is no denying that birth is initially a stressful event for all babies. Thankfully, the hormones a baby secretes during labour (such as vasopressin) help to dampen the impact of this stress and even function as a mild painkiller.[1]

Research among maternity-care providers has found that most believe the birth experience has a direct impact on newborn behaviour, such as increasing or decreasing levels of fussiness.[2] These professionals believe babies who have calmer births are calmer in temperament.

So what can we do to provide a calmer birthing environment for babies?

- Keep the room warm.
- Consider dimming lights at the moment of birth and for the first hour or two afterwards.
- Minimise handling by others.

- Choose soft clothing and blankets.

- Delay wiping and bathing.

- Have as much skin-to-skin contact as possible.

Calm newborn environments aren't restricted to a specific type of birth. You can make the world more comforting and calming for your baby no matter how or where they are born.

What is skin-to-skin contact — and why is it so important?

Skin-to-skin contact — the act of holding your naked baby against your own naked skin — is, perhaps, the most powerful tool in nature for calming them and helping their body systems to stabilise. When a baby is in direct skin contact with their parents, it helps them to relax and has numerous physiological benefits, including:[3]

- better chance of successful breastfeeding initiation

- increased duration of breastfeeding

- more stable breathing

- more stable heart rate

- better blood-glucose (sugar) levels

- better temperature regulation.

Skin-to-skin contact is easy to instigate after almost any type of birth. If the room is cool, make sure you use a soft blanket to cover the baby's back, with their torso in contact with yours.

PARENTING Q&A

Q. *What causes that distinct newborn smell?*
A. *That smell comes from the vernix that covers the baby's skin at birth. Interestingly, research shows that the smell triggers a part of the adult brain related to feelings of pleasure and reward; that's why so many say that the scent of a newborn is addictive.*[4]

The breast crawl (the innate drive to feed)

When a baby is born and placed prone (tummy down) on their mother's belly or chest, they instinctively begin to crawl, or rather slowly shuffle, towards her breasts. They will slowly begin to pull their knees up under them and use their feet to propel themselves upwards. The movement is tiny – with the baby covering only about 5cm in the hour it usually takes for the breast crawl to be completed – but purposeful.[5] The

Anthropology Titbit In Latin America, the tradition of '*la cuarentena*' (or quarantine) encourages new mothers to spend forty days at home focusing on their babies, bonding, establishing breastfeeding and healing their bodies after childbirth. During this time, they are cared for by female relatives, and while some foods are encouraged (such as soups), others are forbidden (those considered too spicy or heavy, for example). Sex is also forbidden in this period, while the mother recovers and recuperates.

FUN FACT
Research using breast pads soaked in either the mother's breast milk or that of another mother has shown that newborns spend more time turning to face the pad containing the milk of their own mother than that of the stranger.[6]

baby is drawn to the mother's breasts by the distinct colour difference of her nipples and areola from the rest of the breast tissue, an increased body temperature in the areola area (up to two degrees warmer than surrounding skin)[7] and the scent of the mother's milk. When babies are allowed to breast crawl and self-attach to the breast (rather than being picked up and actively positioned at the breast) the initiation of breastfeeding is usually easier.

The fontanelles (why your baby looks like Mr Spock)

In the previous chapter, we briefly touched on the topic of cranial sutures and fontanelles. When babies are born, their skulls are not fused like those of adults. The ability of the skull bones (there are five in total) to overlap means that the baby's head is smaller and easier to birth. Newborns can often have very

Parent Observation 'When our son was born, his head was such a strange shape – it almost looked like an ice-cream cone. I was worried that there was something wrong, but the midwives reassured us that it was normal and would return to a round shape quickly, which it did.'

strange, elongated heads, but in the days following birth, their cranial bones will return to their usual position, encouraged by the movement of their jaw when they suckle and feed, which helps to pull the bones into place – just one of the reasons why it is so important not to time or restrict feeds in the newborn weeks. The fontanelles – the soft, boneless spots in your baby's head, allow their skull to grow quickly, giving space for the developing brain inside. The posterior fontanelle (at the back of the head) will usually close by the time they are two or three months old, while the anterior fontanelle (at the front – the one that many refer to as a 'soft spot') usually closes by the time the child is eighteen months to two years old.

PARENTING Q&A

Q. *I'm worried about my baby's brain being hurt if we accidentally touch or damage their soft spot. What can we do to protect it?*

A. *Although the soft spot, the anterior fontanelle, is not covered in bone, it is still covered in a tough membrane that protects the baby's brain, so you don't need to worry about everyday handling and touch.*

There is no preparation for the sight of a first child. There should be a song for women to sing in this moment, or a prayer to recite. But perhaps there is none, because there are no words strong enough to name that moment.

Anita Diamant, American author

The magical healing properties of kisses

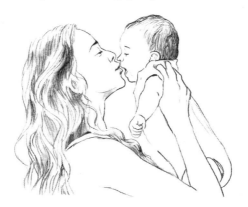

When you hold your baby for the first time, you will probably find yourself automatically kissing their head. This behaviour helps with more than just bonding. When a breastfeeding mother kisses her newborn baby's head she will ingest the pathogens on the baby's skin. The mother's body will then create antibodies to any pathogens she has ingested from the baby. These antibodies are finally secreted in the breast milk that the baby will drink, giving the baby immunity to pathogens they may be carrying. It's an incredibly clever way to help to build the baby's immune system.

FUN FACT
A baby's brain grows 1 per cent each day in the
newborn period.[8]

How the brain develops from birth to three months

At birth, your baby's brain is around a third of the size it will be in adulthood. During their first three months, it will grow rapidly (by 64 per cent), reaching 55 per cent of adult brain size by the time they are three months old.[9] The baby's brain also has at birth all the neurons it will ever have; what it does not have, however, are the connections between them, or synapses. The first three months see a period of major synaptic growth (known as 'exuberance' or 'exuberant synaptogenesis') which continues throughout the first year; some also refer to this period as a 'synaptic big bang'. While many of the developmental changes in the newborn brain happen because of genetic encoding, a sizeable percentage occur because of the environment the baby lives in and the type of care they receive.

The cerebellum – the part of the brain responsible for voluntary movements, co-ordination and balance – is the fastest-growing area of the infant brain, doubling in size in the first three months, reflecting the rapid progress of movement-related skills in newborns. The second-fastest growing area

Neuroscience Nugget It takes between thirty minutes and two hours to complete one synaptic connection in the brain.[10]

How can you encourage optimal brain growth?

You will likely find yourself inundated with adverts from retailers and service providers who promise that their products and classes encourage optimal brain development. The good news is that you don't need to spend any money, or even leave your home for this – because the best way to encourage brain growth and new synaptic connections is simply to spend quality time with your baby. In short, *you* are the greatest brain-development tool in their world.

The following are specific ways to nurture your newborn's brain:

- Lots and lots of cuddles[11]
- Making eye contact with them
- Smiling at them
- Talking to them
- Singing to them
- Dancing and swaying with them

Never underestimate how important you are to your baby's progress or how impactful your everyday interactions with them are.

Neuroscience Nugget The cerebral cortex – the part of the brain responsible for conscious thoughts, actions and feelings – is poorly connected at birth. You may hear some people say that a baby is spoiled by too many hugs or is acting in a manipulative way when they cry to be held, but this is physiologically impossible, as their brain simply isn't mature enough for this sort of thought process.

is the hippocampus – responsible for learning and making memories – which grows 47 per cent in the first three months and reflects the enormous amount of learning that a newborn does; everything in the world is new to them and the level of daily learning about their surroundings, their own body's abilities and also their relationship with you is simply astounding. Their positive interactions with you and the world around them triggers your baby's brain to form new neural connections, or synapses, and the more time you spend with them, the more their brain will grow and develop.

FUN FACT

If a baby's body grew at the same rate as their brain, they would weigh about 77kg by the time they were only one month old.

PARENTING Q&A

Q. *Are there any differences between the male and female brain at birth?*

A. *Recent scientific thinking is that a considerable proportion of neurological differences between males and females in later childhood and adulthood are due to the process of societal conditioning and the intense gender stereotyping babies are exposed to from birth. There are also physical differences between male and female brains at birth, though, with female brains showing more connections in the part responsible for speech and male brains being slightly larger.*

> **FUN FACT**
> When a baby is born via waterbirth, they will automatically hold their breath if they go under water, due to a reflex that all babies have, called the diving reflex, retained from their time in utero.

Physical development from birth to three months

A baby is born with a series of automatic actions that their bodies perform in relation to certain stimuli. These are known as 'primitive reflexes'.

Primitive reflexes (see examples overleaf) originate from the baby's brain stem – the part of the brain responsible for the automatic functions the body needs for survival. They are only present for the first three to four months of a baby's life, after which they will be suppressed as the part of the brain in charge of voluntary movement matures.

The following are some primitive reflexes you may notice in your newborn.

Moro reflex

Often known as the startle reflex, this occurs when you place your baby down, they hear a loud noise or something else that startles them and they fling their arms and legs out and up in the air briefly as a response, before bringing them back in again. This is often accompanied by crying.

Palmar grasp reflex

This is a cute reflex that many new parents mistake for their baby consciously holding their finger in an act of love. In fact,

FUN FACT

A baby can trigger the Moro reflex when they are startled by their own cries or passing wind.

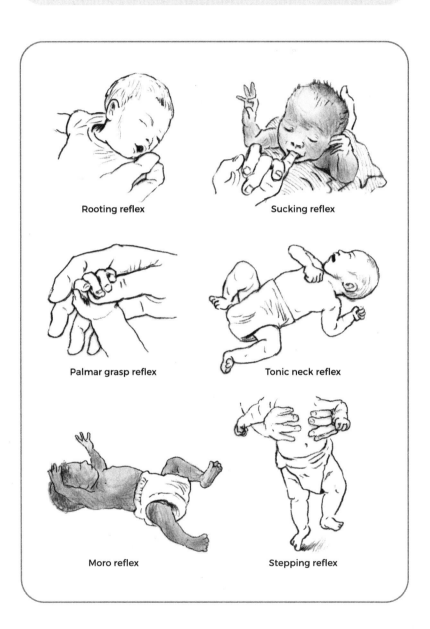

Rooting reflex

Sucking reflex

Palmar grasp reflex

Tonic neck reflex

Moro reflex

Stepping reflex

when their palms are stroked it triggers a grasping reflex in newborns, and they will close their fingers around yours.

Rooting reflex

When your baby's cheeks or the corners of their mouths are gently touched, they will rapidly move their head from side to side and open their mouth, enabling them to latch onto a breast or a bottle.

Sucking reflex

When something touches your newborn's mouth, they will open their lips and suck on it – whatever it is!

Stepping reflex

When your baby is held gently around their torso and their feet touch a firm surface, they will lift their feet up and down in a stepping motion that mimics a walking movement.

Tonic-neck reflex

When your baby turns their head to one side, this reflex (sometimes called 'the fencing reflex' because it looks as if the baby is making a fencing pose) will cause the arm on the side that the head is turned to straighten and the other arm to bend.

Physical milestones

It will seem as if your baby changes daily in the first few months – which, of course, they do – but the differences are

Every child begins the world again.
Henry David Thoreau, American philosopher

most striking in the newborn period. Physically, they will grow around 2.5cm in length per month and will usually gain 0.6–0.9kg in weight per month. This is also a period of rapid motor development, or what is more commonly referred to as movement-based milestones.

Newborn to one month

In the first month after birth, your baby's movements will seem quite uncontrolled and jerky. This is because their brain still has some maturing to do before they can purposefully control their own body movements. One of the first parts of the body that a baby masters moving consciously is their neck, enabling them to turn their head to the side to feed. They also have some conscious control over their eye muscles (albeit not full control, so don't worry if you see their eyes wandering out-wards), although their vision is still very blurry at this point, and they can only focus on things around 20–25cm away from their face. A newborn's eyes are exceptionally light sensitive, and they will often close them when exposed to bright light. They can discern between black and white, hence they are drawn to black and white contrasting images, the first colour they can see being red.

Your baby can hear fairly well in the first month, although the middle ear is likely to still contain a little fluid after their birth. This will slowly drain away, however. At this age, babies usually respond the most to higher-pitched noises, which is

Anthropology Titbit In Latvia, newborns are bathed in a sauna-type warm environment and massaged with breast milk in a ritual known as *pirtīža*, or 'pushing bristle'. This is said to make babies more content and calmer.

why adults tend to subconsciously raise the pitch of their voice when speaking to them.

One to two months

In the second month of life, your baby is working hard to develop head control; especially when they are lying on their front, they will start to lift their head up clear of the floor a little. Their primitive reflexes are starting to diminish (although they won't fully disappear yet) and their movement starts to become more conscious and purposeful. You will probably notice their movements become more fluid and less jerky, too – another sign that the cerebellum, the part of their brain responsible for conscious movements, is maturing. During this month, you may notice that they move their arms around when they are excited – for instance, when you are playing with them – and many will find their hands towards the end of this period, trying to bring them to their mouths.

When your baby is around six weeks old, you may well catch their first smile. Before this, you will have seen signs of smiling during their sleep, but this is not a conscious smile – rather, it's wind or another reflex-related movement.

Your baby's vision is also maturing, and by the time they turn two months old, you should find that they are able to focus their eyes on you (and on objects). At this point, they will likely be able to see more colours, although experts are

Parent Observation 'The first time she smiled at me, when she was a month and a half old, made all of the tiredness and the hard work worth it! I felt like she thought, I think Mum really needs some inspiration today, so she flashed me a big grin. It worked!'

> **FUN FACT**
>
> *By the second month, a baby can distinguish their mother's voice from that of a stranger. When they hear their mother talking, their brain responds in a different way from when they hear a stranger.*[12]

unsure if they can discern between different shades, so they will be drawn to colours that are highly contrasting. Their vision should be mature enough by this age that they are able to recognise you – just in time to give you your first smile!

Tummy time

When your baby spends time lying on their front (commonly known as 'tummy time'), it helps many different parts of their body:

- It builds strong back and neck muscles.
- It encourages development of the hip and leg muscles, ready for crawling.
- It helps with good posture and spinal alignment.
- It helps to prevent plagiocephaly – otherwise known as flattening of the skull.
- It strengthens their arms, which aids with reaching, crawling and pulling up as they grow.

Tummy time is also good for babies who suffer with wind and constipation, as the gentle pressure on their belly can help to provide relief.

Ideally, your baby will spend a couple of minutes on their tummy several times a day, from birth. A number of shorter sessions are usually tolerated more than one or two longer ones, but as they get more used to it, you can build up the time spent on their tummy. You should only do tummy time when your baby is awake, and you should always be with them to supervise. You may find using a special tummy-time cushion is more comfortable for them. You can also lie on the floor on your back and encourage them to lie on their tummy on top of you – the natural curves of your body will provide support, your warmth will help to calm them and being able to look into each other's eyes should help them to feel more settled. If this doesn't work, then try lying on the floor on your tummy yourself opposite your baby, so that they can look into your eyes. Carrying them in a sling or carrier, facing in – tummy to tummy – can also provide a form of tummy time.

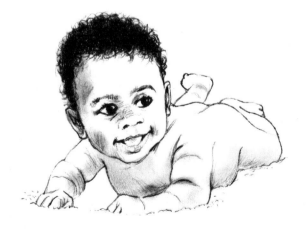

FUN FACT

By the age of three months, babies are able to recognise their mothers in photographs. When shown a picture of their mother or a stranger, a baby spends significantly more time looking at the one of their mother.[13]

Growth charts and centiles

When you visit your health visitor or family doctor, they will weigh and measure your baby and plot their weight and height on something known as a growth – or centile – chart. This helps to check that their growth is following an expected trajectory. Different charts are used for boys and girls, as their growth is slightly different.

The health professionals who plot your baby's growth will be looking to see that they stick roughly to a centile. Short for percentile, centiles are lines of expected growth, compared to that of other babies. So, for instance, if your baby follows the seventy-fifth centile for height, this means they are taller than 75 per cent of other babies. If they are on the fortieth centile for weight, this means they weigh less than 60 per cent of other babies. Do remember that it is natural for some babies to be smaller and some bigger than others. Just like adults, nobody is the same – we are all wonderfully unique. What matters more than the actual centile they are on is that your baby's growth roughly follows an expected line for their centile, rather than shooting up or dropping off dramatically.

FUN FACT
The first two emotions your baby is likely to feel are stress,
or tension, and calmness, or a feeling of being relaxed.
It is believed that babies feel these two distinct emotions
by the time they are three months old.

In their second month, babies become more interested in sounds, particularly talking, and they will often quieten and listen to the sound of voices.

Two to three months

From two to three months of age your baby will look quite different to the curled-up newborn you held in your arms only a few weeks before. You will notice that their movements are now controlled and purposeful and they will have much more muscle tone. Head control continues to improve, and at three months, babies may be able to prop themselves up on their arms when they are in a prone position (on their tummies).

By three months of age, your baby may be able to bring their hands together; they will also likely open their hands more, rather than keeping them in the curled-fist hold that they had in the newborn weeks. Many babies of this age enjoy entertaining themselves by opening and closing their hands, as well as actively kicking their legs when laid on their backs and digging their feet into the floor when on their fronts. Along with developing head control and core strength, these movements are all important precursors to crawling.

Finally, your baby's eyesight continues to progress, and images become far less blurry as their distance vision improves.

Feeding and eating from birth to three months

When the baby is in utero, they receive all the nutrients they need from the placenta; once they are born, the placenta's job is taken over by milk. Breast milk, or infant formula milk, provides everything your newborn needs nutritionally at this age, and also fulfils their thirst needs.

How much milk does your baby need?

At birth, your baby's stomach is tiny, and holds around one teaspoon of milk. If they are breastfed, they will receive all the nutrients they need from the small amounts of colostrum (the first milk produced by mothers that is thick, yellowish and higher in fat than normal breast milk) for the first couple of days. By Day 2, a newborn's stomach holds up to a table-

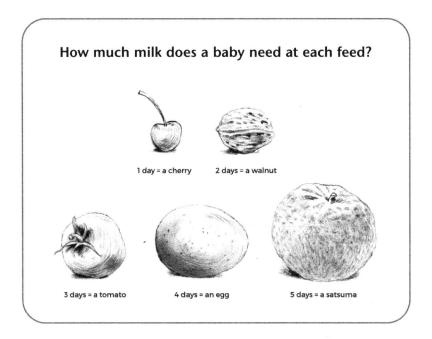

How much milk does a baby need at each feed?

1 day = a cherry   2 days = a walnut

3 days = a tomato   4 days = an egg   5 days = a satsuma

spoon of milk, and this doubles by Day 3. By Day 4, the baby's stomach holds three tablespoons of milk and by Day 5, this increases to five. By the time your baby is a month old, their stomach can hold up to 150ml milk – or ten tablespoons' worth.

A formula-fed baby will usually consume between 150 and 200ml of milk per kilogram of their weight daily, until they are around six months old, while an exclusively breastfed baby will consume an average of 750ml per day at one month of age.

PARENTING Q&A

Q. *How do I know my breastfed baby has had enough milk?*

A. *In the first couple of days, your baby is likely to only have two or three wet nappies. It is not uncommon for them not to poo for a few days after the initial meconium (the first tar-like poo) is passed. By Day 4, they should have two soft yellow poos a day and more frequent wet nappies. By Day 5, wet nappies should be heavy and happen at least six times per day. You should also be able to see and hear your baby swallowing milk during feeds, and they should be generally content during and after. Frequent feeding in the early days (and nights) is common and not a sign that you are not making enough milk. In fact, this cluster feeding, as it is known, is an important way for your baby to increase your milk supply. If you are concerned about their feeding at all, then speaking to a lactation consultant or breastfeeding counsellor is a good idea. See Resources, page 258, for some organisations that can help.*

How can you tell if your baby is hungry?

It can be hard to tell when your baby is hungry in the early weeks. You will soon learn to spot their signs as you get to know them more, but until you do, early hunger signs to look out for include:

- rooting (moving the head from side to side, as if looking for the nipple – even if your baby is bottle-fed)
- moving their fists to their mouth
- opening and closing their mouth, licking or smacking their lips
- sucking on anything close to their mouths
- fidgeting and squirming.

Later signs of hunger, when your baby is really desperate to feed, include fussiness, crying and very agitated movements.

PARENTING Q&A

Q. *My mum has been telling us to get our daughter into a feeding schedule as soon as possible, but I feel more comfortable feeding her when I think she's hungry. Is that OK?*

A. *Feeding to a timing schedule is an old-fashioned concept, and a lot of recent research has shown it is much healthier for a baby, particularly a newborn, to be fed on demand (following their hunger cues), regardless of whether they are breast- or bottle-fed. Your baby knows when they're hungry or thirsty much better than any chart or table!*

Parent Observation 'When my son was tiny, I could always tell he was getting hungry when he started wriggling around like a little worm and opening and closing his mouth like a baby bird. If I managed to feed him before he cried, it was so much easier than trying to calm him down if he got over-hungry and cried lots. So I soon learned to watch him like a hawk.'

FUN FACT
The temperature of amniotic fluid is between 36.5 and 37°C, so a newborn will never have swallowed cold fluid before. Breast milk is an average of 37°C – hence why babies are usually happier to drink warmed milk if they are bottle feeding.

Sleep development from birth to three months

Newborns sleep a lot, although their sleep patterns are vastly different to ours. As adults, we tend to sleep in fewer blocks of a couple of hours, whereas newborns sleep in many tiny blocks of around half an hour. So it's likely you will find that your newborn's sleep patterns clash quite a bit with your own sleep needs. While you are biologically primed to sleep all night, your newborn will wake just as much during the night as they do during the day, often more so, as the quiet and stillness of night make them feel less safe and secure. Conversely, in the daytime, you may be desperate to play with your baby or introduce them to friends and family, and it can be frustrating

FUN FACT
Newborn babies sleep for between sixteen and eighteen hours
in every twenty-four-hour period. They sleep so much because
they need to conserve energy for growing and
brain development.

when they sleep through everything. But don't worry – this daytime sleepiness won't last for ever, just as the sleepless nights won't either (however never-ending they may feel).

Newborns have four main stages of consciousness:

Asleep

1) Quiet sleep: this is a deeper sleep state, where the baby will be noticeably quiet and still. This stage is also known as nREM (non-rapid eye movement) sleep. Your newborn will spend around 50 per cent of their time asleep in this state.

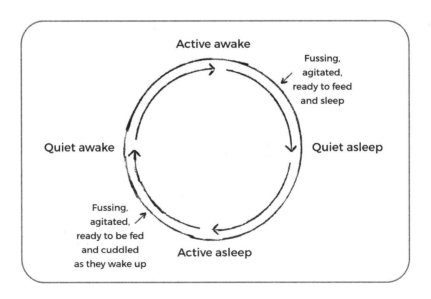

2) Active sleep: this is a light sleep state, during which you will notice fluttering eyelids, grimacing, grunting, changeable breathing patterns and small body movements. This stage is also known as REM (rapid eye movement) sleep. Your newborn will spend around 50 per cent of their time asleep in this state.

Awake

3) Quiet awake: during this phase, your baby will be awake and alert, but lying quite still and quietly, staring at certain objects.

4) Active awake: when your baby wakes up a little more, they will be more active in their body, moving around a little, and will more actively look around their environment. Towards the end of this period, they can start to get cranky and fussy. This indicates that they are getting tired and are ready to go to sleep again. Catching them before they get overstimulated and overtired will mean that they will both feed and go to sleep more easily, so try to observe your baby closely during their awake period and see if you can learn their cues for when their active awake period needs to transition into sleep.

Neuroscience Nugget Research has found that the twitches your baby makes during sleep help their brain learn to co-ordinate their bodily movements.[14] Adults usually only twitch during the active phase of sleep, but newborns twitch in quiet sleep, too, indicating there is a lot more happening in their brains when they sleep.

FUN FACT

Your baby won't be able to tell the difference between night and day until they are around three months old. This is because their circadian rhythm (body clock) is underdeveloped and their brains do not secrete the hormones of sleep and waking (melatonin and cortisol, respectively) to a pattern of night and day in the way that our brains do. So, for the newborn period, don't fret about teaching them the difference between night and day because it won't make a difference. It's a purely biological change and the only real thing you can do is wait. You should see a pattern emerging slowly when they're around ten to twelve weeks old.

Helping your newborn to sleep

Only a short time ago your baby was used to being held tightly by a warm uterus twenty-four hours a day. Up until birth, they have never been alone. They have also never experienced light, air, changing noises and smells, or clothing, cold or hard surfaces. It makes sense, then, that the environment that keeps them calm and helps them to sleep the most is one which mimics life in utero – or, as I call it, their 'womb world'. This concept is also referred to as 'the fourth trimester' (see page 25).

Womb	World
Dark	Light
Muffled sounds	Loud noises
Constant warm temperature	Fluctuating temperatures
Constant nutrition	Hunger and thirst

Confined space	Lots of space
Aquatic	Air
Inability to smell	Many different smells
Constant contact with mother	Dramatically reduced contact
Constantly 'held'	Held far less
Naked	Clothed
All surroundings soft and warm	Many surroundings hard and cold

So how can you replicate your baby's womb world for them in the fourth trimester?

- Hold them in your arms or in a sling or baby carrier, as much as possible – and 'wear' them facing inwards.
- Gently sway or dance with them to replicate the movement they would have felt in utero.
- Choose soft clothing, with no waistbands, zips, buttons or other things that may dig into their skin.
- Use a swaddle wrap – but only if they are under ten weeks of age and are unable to roll onto their front in their sleep.
- Encourage skin-to-skin contact – sit and hold them facing inwards on your bare chest for hugs, with a warm blanket over their back.
- Warm baths (body temperature – around 36–37°C); you could also get in with them if there is somebody else to help you to get in and out.

Parent Observation 'My newborn used to fall asleep within moments of being driven in the car. I always wondered if the noise of the engine and the motion made them remember being in the womb.'

- Play white-noise recordings or recordings of household noises, such as tumble dryers, hoovers and hairdryers.
- Go for a drive in the car; the rumble and hum of the engine can mimic noises in utero.

FUN FACT

Newborns have underdeveloped hearing – it is not as discerning as that of an adult, and they struggle to tell the difference between background noises and human voices. So often, the sound of a hairdryer or white noise can reassure them as much as you talking to them, if not more so.

Anthropology Titbit In Japan, most babies sleep in the same bed (or futon) as their parents (a practice known as bedsharing), rather than in a crib or a cot alone.[15] Interestingly, the Japanese have one of the lowest SIDS (cot death) rates in the world.

My favourite time, when I look back from day one with my sons and with, obviously, my daughter – each parent talks about the waking up during the night and the feeding during the night but, for me, that was the most special time. It doesn't matter what time of the night it is or how tired you are, they make you smile, they make you happy.
David Beckham, English footballer

What is colic?

Colic is diagnosed when a baby cries for more than three hours per day, more than three days per week. It is not actually a disease or disorder, but a medical label used for unsettled babies. Trying to find the underlying cause of the baby being so unhappy is the best course of action, especially considering that popular colic remedies sold in pharmacies, containing an ingredient called simethicone, are no more effective than a placebo. Common causes of unsettled newborns include not understanding the womb-to-world transition; following sleeping and feeding schedules, rather than the baby's cues; feeding issues, such as a tongue tie or difficulty latching; discomfort from the birth, and an imbalance in the baby's gut flora – or 'good bacteria' (known as the microbiome). Research has shown that infant probiotics, which work to reintroduce these 'good bacteria', can have a positive impact on colic.[16]

PARENTING Q&A

Q. *I've been told I shouldn't rush to pick up my baby, otherwise they won't be able to self-soothe. Is this true?*

A. *This is a very outdated way of thinking. Newborns are incapable of self-soothing, and scientists have found that the best way to help them with this skill is to respond to their needs.[17] So pick your baby up whenever you need to, safe in the knowledge that your responsiveness is helping them with self-regulation skills.*

Keeping your baby safe while they sleep

- Your baby should always be put to sleep on their back.
- If your baby is in a cot or crib, put them down at the bottom with their feet to the foot of the cot/crib.
- Don't use baby sleep positioners or nests while your baby is unsupervised.
- Don't use cot or crib bumpers.
- Don't leave any toys or other loose items in the cot or crib.
- Make sure your baby doesn't overheat; keep blankets to lighter layers or use a baby sleeping bag up to 2.5 togs in weight.
- Only share a bed with your baby if you have made a conscious decision to do so and you follow the safety guidelines below. Be careful to not accidentally fall asleep with them in the bed, in a nursing chair or on a sofa.
- Only share a bed with your baby if they are healthy, were not born prematurely and you are breastfeeding. If you are formula-feeding, opt for a co-sleeper (open-sided) crib next to you instead.
- Only share a bed with your baby if you are not taking any medication that makes you drowsy, you have not drunk any alcohol and you are a non-smoker.
- If bedsharing, the baby should only sleep next to their mother on the outside of the bed, sleeping at breast height (lower than any pillows) with the mother making a protective frame shape around the baby (see illustration opposite).
- Do not share a bed with your baby if they are swaddled. If you use a swaddle wrap and the baby is

in a cot or crib, make sure to stop using the swaddle before they can roll onto their tummy.

• You baby should spend all their time sleeping (both for naps in the day and at night) in the same room as you.

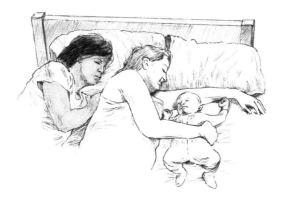

PARENTING Q&A

Q. *Is it safe for my baby to sleep in their own room if we use a video baby monitor and a breathing sensor?*

A. *Unfortunately, not. Many parents believe their baby is safe sleeping alone if they use a breathing sensor or monitor, but these provide false reassurance and do not reduce the rate of SIDS (cot death). Babies should spend all their sleeping time in the same room as you, not only because of your supervision, but also because when you breathe and exhale carbon dioxide, this triggers the baby to inhale. If you are not in the same room as them, this protective gaseous exchange process doesn't happen.*

When your baby's sleep isn't normal

Although it is normal for babies to wake regularly through the night, sometimes waking can be extreme and accompanied by unsettled and fractious behaviour. Here are some common causes of extremely difficult sleep in babies:

- Gastroesophageal reflux disease (GORD) – where the sphincter (muscle ring) in the oesophagus (food pipe) is not mature and allows food to travel back up, usually causing frequent vomiting. However, sometimes it can be known as 'silent reflux', where all the symptoms are present minus the vomiting.

- Tongue tie – where the piece of skin that holds the tongue to the base of the mouth (the frenulum) is too tight, causing the baby to struggle with feeding (see picture below).

- Latch problems – where the baby struggles to feed well (from the breast or bottle), perhaps because of a tongue tie, a lip tie (where the lip is held too tightly to the gum, meaning it struggles to flare out

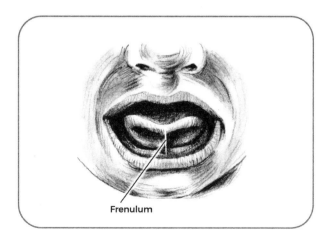

Frenulum

appropriately to get a good seal during a feed) or other positional issues.

- Discomfort – the baby may be experiencing some muscular tightness from the birth causing distress when they lie in certain positions.
- Enlarged adenoids – when the adenoids (small tissue lumps at the back of the nose, forming part of the immune system) are swollen, this can cause difficulties with breathing, which can impact sleep.
- Allergies – such as cow's milk protein allergy (CMPA) can cause gastrointestinal and other discomfort, which can impact sleep.

If you feel instinctively that your baby's sleep is outside of the realms of normality for their age and you feel that they are quite unsettled, then do speak to your family doctor, health visitor, lactation consultant or breastfeeding counsellor (see Resources, page 258).

Social and psychological development from birth to three months

While a newborn baby may not appear to be interacting socially – they don't yet smile and they can't hold a verbal conversation – they are actually highly social from the moment

FUN FACT
A newborn can anticipate being picked up and will stiffen and hold their muscles in a specific way when they sense that their parents or carers are about to lift them.

Neuroscience Nugget Research has shown that the more nurturance a baby receives in infancy, the more the area of their brain responsible for socialisation grows in later life.[18]

of birth. Young babies are able to attract the attention of their parents and carers through crying, body movements and something as simple as holding their gaze. Similarly, they are incredibly responsive to the movements, speech and eye contact of their parents and carers.

The newborn period is all about your baby learning to trust you and forming attachments. The best way to do this? Cuddle them, talk to them, sing to them and respond to their needs as quickly as you are able to.

What is reciprocity?

Reciprocity is a term used to describe an exchange of communication between parent, or other adults, and child by tuning in to the baby's emotions through their verbal and non-verbal cues and adjusting the way they behave and connect accordingly. For instance, if an adult is playing with a baby and the baby is happy, the adult will interpret their behaviour as a sign that the play should continue. If the baby starts to cry, or looks tired or uncomfortable, the adult will cease the play and pick the baby up for a cuddle. And the baby grasps the adult's actions and communication, too. Research shows that parents who score highly in reciprocity raise children who are more sociable and have better relationships with others as they grow.[19]

Being touched and caressed, being massaged, is food for the infant; food as necessary as minerals, vitamins and proteins.
Frederick Leboyer, French obstetrician

Touch – the greatest calming and communication tool

One of the ways in which we can communicate love to a newborn and help them to feel calmer and more relaxed is through touch. When you touch your baby's skin with gentle strokes and massage, they, and you, release a hormone called oxytocin which helps you to bond. Research also shows that massaging them regularly helps to improve their sleep, reduces symptoms of colic and the amount that they cry and lowers their levels of the stress hormone, cortisol.[20] Regular infant massage can also help your baby to grow and improve their immune system, decreasing the number of illnesses that they get.

Language and communication development from birth to three months

Crying is your newborn's biggest form of communication at this stage, but although they are not yet talking, there are plenty of other ways they will connect with you over

FUN FACT
Babies prefer looking at faces, compared to any other shapes, from birth. Just another indicator that they are hard-wired for socialisation and connection.

the coming weeks, including smiling and mimicking your behaviour and movements. One of the earliest ways babies learn to (eventually) talk is by watching your mouth movements and mimicking them. They also learn how to take turns in conversations through the early verbal interactions they have with you. This is why it is so important to talk to your baby regularly and allow them to see your face as much as possible – for instance, by choosing a pram or buggy that can be used 'parent-facing' rather than forward-facing.

When you talk to your baby, try to avoid background noise (such as having the television on all day), so they will be able to focus more on your voice, which will help language development. You may also consider reading to them a little every day; it's never too early for this and it can really help their language skills.

PARENTING Q&A

Q. *Sometimes I can't work out why my baby is crying. How do I learn what to do to help?*

A. *You're not alone – every parent struggles to understand their baby at times. Over the coming months, you will gradually begin to interpret your baby's cries and come to understand what they need most of the time, but in the early days, it can be confusing. A lot of the time cries can be soothed by picking the baby up and cuddling them, or offering them a feed; but in times when this doesn't work, you can be assured that even if you can't stop their tears, the fact that you are holding them will help to protect their brain from any of the toxic effects of prolonged crying.[21]*

Play ideas for babies from birth to three months

Play is the primary tool for development and learning at all ages, even the newborn months. Play helps to build relationships, to feel connected to you and to show them that they are important to you and worth your time.

Suggested play activities at this age include:

- singing nursery rhymes
- making silly faces and sounds
- dancing together
- blowing raspberries
- counting their fingers and toes.

Picking the best time to play with your baby

The best time to play with your baby is when they are moving from a state of quiet awake to a state of active awake (see page 49), and then throughout the period of active awake that they are happy and content. Be sure to watch for signs of overstimulation, such as deliberately averting their gaze, yawning, getting fidgety and beginning to cry. It may be tempting to try to cheer your baby up at this point to encourage more play, but it's much better to see these as signs that they have finished with playing and now need to feed and sleep. They only need very short bursts of play – around ten to fifteen minutes at a time.

Recommended toys

- **Black and white cloth books,** or pictures, for them to look at
- **Dangling objects** they can look at and eventually reach for, such as mobiles
- **A soft floor mat** – to allow them to move their body freely without the confines of a crib or pram
- **A tummy-time mat** – a special mat that helps to support them while they lie on their tummy
- **A blanket or similar piece of fabric,** such as a taggy blanket, with different textures for them to feel

Remember, newborns cannot discern subtle colour shades (such as pastels) and find it more interesting to look at strong, bright contrasting ones, or black and white. Choosing toys with this in mind will encourage more interest.

The newborn months really are fleeting. One day you will look at your baby and realise quite how much they have changed in such a short space of time. Now isn't the time to dwell on the past, though; rather, it's time to get excited about the months to come, when they will develop more in both body and mind, and to enjoy wondering what new skills they will soon master. The next chapter will help you to do just this, as we cover the incredible things they will achieve from three to six months.

3

Three to Six Months

Your baby has changed so much in the last three months. Sometimes it can feel as if time is speeding by, leaving you struggling to catch your breath, as they rapidly grow and develop, learning new skills weekly. Wasn't it only yesterday that they were curled on your chest, barely bigger than the two hands you used to gently hold them? Now they greet you with big grins, their body is so much stronger and their movements clearly purposeful. But it doesn't end here – three to six months is another period of huge growth, both physically and emotionally. Let's look at some of the major ways you can expect your baby to change over this three-month period.

How the brain develops from three to six months

Your baby's brain is still growing dramatically during this period. At three months, it is around 55 per cent of the size of an adult's brain and continues to grow during this period at a rate of around 0.4 per cent every single day.

The three-to-six-month period brings the hippocampus to the forefront (this is the part of the brain responsible for learning and memory). Of course, physical development is still important at this age, with more controlled and conscious

Neuroscience Nugget While your baby's brain growth in utero was largely determined by genetics, now the majority of it is determined by their interactions with you and their environment. What is the best way to encourage optimal brain development? Love, nurturance, lots of hugs and speaking to your baby.

movements appearing, and the cerebellum continues to grow at a staggering rate. So you will continue to notice rapid physical changes during this period, but you will also see a dramatic leap in social and communication skills.

Research has shown that by six months of age, a baby already understands the facial expressions of others and can attribute emotions (happiness and anger, for example) to them.[1] By four months of age, they appear to recognise their own name when spoken, and by five months, they understand that it is used as a way to gain their attention and will turn towards the person speaking it.[2]

Many cognitive psychologists see the brain as a computer. But every single brain is absolutely individual, both in its development and in the way it experiences the world.
Gerald Edelman, American biologist

Neuroscience Nugget The visual cortex (the part of the brain responsible for sight) sees peak synapse production between four and eight months of age.

PARENTING Q&A

Q. *Is there such a thing as developmental leaps?*

A. *Sadly not. While it would be lovely to have a definitive timeline of how your baby will behave based upon 'leaps' of neurological development, this is not reflected in the evidence base. Indeed, the robust evidence that we do have indicates that brain development occurs over a range of different ages and is unique for each baby. While parents and carers may note specific behaviours at certain ages that align with a 'leap', it is likely that these are a bit of a self-fulfilling prophecy – a little like astrology: if you expect to see something, you are more likely to notice it.*

Synaptogenesis – the creation of new synapses, or connections, in your baby's brain – continues to be the emphasis during this period. Many more synapses are made than the baby will end up needing or using at this age, but a later process of pruning will remove any extra unwanted ones.

Physical development from three to six months

By the time your baby is four months old, they will likely have doubled their birth weight. Physical milestones are rapidly acquired during this period, reflecting the huge amount that's going on in the area of the brain responsible for conscious movement control, as well as improved vision and muscle strength.

> **FUN FACT**
> *Babies don't secrete tears when they cry until they are one month old. In the newborn period, their tear ducts only produce enough liquid to moisturise their eyes, so their tears are 'dry'.*

Physical milestones

From three months of age, babies become increasingly engaged with the world around them, thanks to a combination of maturing vision and more motor skills allowing them to interact more actively. Let's take a look at the specific milestones that occur during this period.

Three to four months

During this period, your baby is working on their physical dexterity. They may start to rock from side to side when they are lying on a flat surface; this movement is an important precursor to rolling. Your baby is also likely to show a growing interest in their hands and will spend a lot of time bringing them up to their mouth and sucking on their fists. Many parents misinterpret this as hunger or teething, but it's a common behaviour that rarely indicates anything other than a fascination with their hands and a growing level of

> **FUN FACT**
> *Babies sneeze more than adults. While we are accustomed to blowing our noses to clear mucus and debris, a baby achieves the same result by sneezing.*

conscious movement. Head control will be a focus, too, at this point, and you will probably find that your baby has much more neck strength than they did just a month ago and is able to hold their head steady for longer.

Around this time you will notice your baby becoming more interested in the world around them. They may turn their head to look at unexpected and loud noises and will probably be experimenting with making different sounds, such as cooing, gurgling and grunting. This is all important practice for learning to speak.

Vision-wise, their eyesight has improved since birth, and they can see more clearly and further away. By the end of this period, they will be developing something known as 'binocular vision', meaning that both eyes will be working together to produce one image. If you imagine looking through a pair of binoculars, you are actually seeing two different images (one through each eyepiece), but your brain works to converge these into one. Binocular vision is acquired from the process of your baby looking around them more as they grow, combined with strengthening eye muscles.

Four to five months

Between four and five months, most babies will have enough head control that when they are lying on their tummies, they

---

FUN FACT

Scientists believe that babies look and sound purposefully cute in order to appeal to all of our senses so that we take care of them.[3] Your baby's big eyes, long eyelashes, yummy smell and beautiful soft, podgy limbs are apparently nature's way of ensuring that they stay safe and encourage us to protect them.

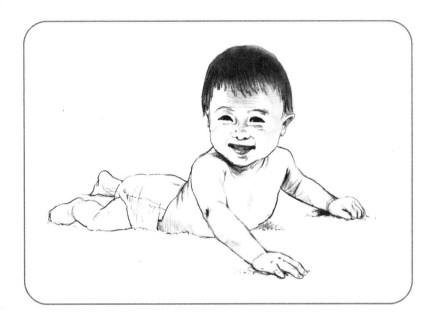

will be able to lift both head and chest clear of the floor, holding themselves up on their elbows and forearms.

You may find that your baby will also roll over for the first time during this month, usually from their back to their tummy (tummy to back takes a little more practice).

At some point between four and five months, babies develop something known as 'perceptual constancy'.[4] This happens when they are able to discern something that may slightly alter the way it looks in different environments. For instance, recognising a toy at night in dim lighting, where details are hard to spot, as being the same toy that they see in

FUN FACT
Babies have almost one hundred more bones than adults.
It takes until toddlerhood for these to begin to
fuse together.

> **Parent Observation** 'My daughter developed a strange grunting noise when she was about five months old that she used to make if she was bored or wanted to be picked up. We're not sure if she learned to make the noise because we picked her up when she did, or if she knew to make the noise to get us to pick her up – either way it worked!'

full detail during the daytime in bright lighting. In the first three to four months of life, babies notice these changes and perceive the objects to be entirely different objects.

Babbling becomes more purposeful at this age, and you will likely notice your baby making sounds deliberately, perhaps to draw your attention to them, or to indicate discomfort or frustration.

Five to six months

Between the ages of five and six months, babies get great enjoyment from making things happen in the world around them, such as pressing buttons to make a noise. Babies learn through

---

PARENTING Q&A

Q. *I always try to put my baby down to sleep on his back, but he almost instantly rolls onto his tummy. Is this OK?*

A. *It's OK for your baby to roll onto their tummy if they do it naturally. Just make sure that you always put them down to sleep on their back. Also, make sure that you stop swaddling as soon as you notice they can roll (if you haven't already).*

repetition, so you can expect them to repeat this behaviour again and again. This is also the age when most babies will reach for toys; this occurs because of a combination of physical development and refinement of their motor skills, but also because their eyesight is more mature, with the beginnings of depth perception appearing at around six months and their vision clarity now being similar to that of an adult (or 20/20 vision). This allows them to judge how far away something is and helps them to learn how far to reach. By this stage, colour vision is similar to that of an adult.

PARENTING Q&A

Q. *Why do babies put everything in their mouths? My five-month-old puts everything he can get his hands on straight into his mouth. I'm worried he is in pain, or he's always hungry.*

A. *Babies learn about the properties of objects through the sensory experience of how they feel in their mouths. This is also a common age for them to play with their hands near their mouths and to move anything they may grab hold of near to their mouths. It isn't necessarily a sign of either teething or hunger.*

Anthropology Titbit Research studying the 48,000-year-old tooth of a Neanderthal baby has suggested that babies back then were weaned onto solid food between five and six months of age[5] – similar to the age at which babies eat their first solid foods today.

When do babies start teething?

Most babies will cut their first tooth between five and seven months of age: it is usually the lower central incisor – in the middle of the bottom jaw. The chart below shows the average age you can expect to see your baby's teeth appearing.

Although many believe that babies show teething symptoms for weeks on end, research indicates that most babies only have genuine symptoms for an average of four days before a tooth appears – the day it arrives and three days afterwards.[6] Many of the symptoms attributed to teething (disrupted nights, drooling, chewing on their hands and irritability) are developmentally normal behaviours for this age.

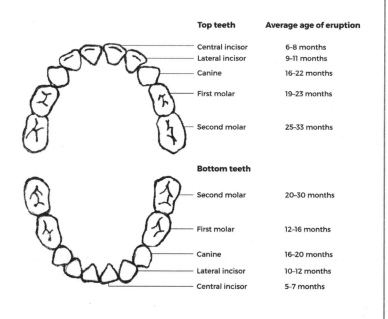

Top teeth	Average age of eruption
Central incisor	6–8 months
Lateral incisor	9–11 months
Canine	16–22 months
First molar	19–23 months
Second molar	25–33 months

Bottom teeth	
Second molar	20–30 months
First molar	12–16 months
Canine	16–20 months
Lateral incisor	10–12 months
Central incisor	5–7 months

Your baby may now be able to roll both ways and you may see their first crawling-related movements, such as rocking and bringing their knees up underneath them when they are on their stomach.

Babbling now takes on more of the sounds of language, such as vowels and consonants, rather than just coos and gurgles.

Feeding and eating from three to six months

When babies are born, they only recognise sweet and sour tastes and don't react to salt. Between the ages of three and four months, however, they begin to recognise and show a preference for saltier tastes.[7] Although we need to consume a small amount of sodium each day, your baby will get all they need from breast or formula milk.

A change in taste buds isn't the only thing that is happening regarding feeding at this age. Several things will need to

PARENTING Q&A

Q. *My baby is twenty weeks old and very interested in watching us eat. He will often try to grab food from my plate. Does this mean he's ready to start eating solids?*

A. *It's unlikely that this is a sign your baby is ready to start solids yet – partly because his gastrointestinal system is still maturing and he won't be able to fully digest the food, but also because this is a common age for babies to start observing others, grabbing anything they can and instantly putting it in their mouths.*

> *FUN FACT*
> *Babies have almost twice as many taste buds as adults.*
> *During infancy, these are constantly being replaced, but the*
> *regeneration stops as we approach adulthood.*

happen in your baby's gastrointestinal system before they are ready to eat solids foods, as follows:

- They will start to secrete more salivary amylase, an enzyme which helps them to digest starch. By six months, levels are similar to those of an adult.
- They will start to secrete more bile salts and lipase as their livers mature, in anticipation of digesting more lipid- (fat-) containing foods
- Their microbiome (the good bacteria) will be continuing to mature and establish itself, influenced heavily by the baby's consumption of oligosaccharides (a simple sugar carbohydrate) from milk.

Your baby's digestive system will be sufficiently mature to fully digest their first solid foods at around six months. (We will cover weaning onto solids more in the next chapter.)

Sleep development from three to six months

You are likely to notice big changes in your baby's sleep during this period. Sadly, though, these changes are often not the move to 'sleeping through the night' that most parents hope for. Let's take a look at what you can expect.

> **FUN FACT**
> *Three- to six-month-old babies spend 50 per cent of their sleep in REM, compared to the 20 to 25 per cent REM sleep that adults get.*

Sleep at three to four months

Once babies turn three months old, a pattern begins to emerge with longer stretches occurring both during the day and at night. Daytime naps also decrease in frequency, with most babies napping between three and five times per day, and each nap lasting anywhere between thirty and sixty minutes.

In total, most three- to four-month-olds will have between fourteen and fifteen hours' sleep in a twenty-four-hour period, around 75 per cent of which takes place at night, indicating that their circadian rhythms (body clocks) are developing, and their bodies are now starting to tell the difference between day and night.[8]

Almost half of all three-month-olds still regularly wake every night – on average 2.7 times.

Sleep at four to five months

Frustratingly, many four-month-old babies experience slightly worse sleep than they did only a month earlier. This can be confusing for parents and carers who may be expecting sleep to continue to improve as the baby gets older; however, temporary dips in sleep, with more waking and less predictability, are usual throughout infancy.[9] At four months, there is rapid development in the visual cortex of the brain, and it

Cat naps

A lot of parents worry about cat naps (naps that are short in length), but they are entirely normal and not a problem – for your baby, that is. Naps in the first six months are commonly short, lasting between 30 and 60 minutes. As babies get older and they take fewer naps per day, their naps usually lengthen, but some babies remain cat nappers, no matter how many naps they have.

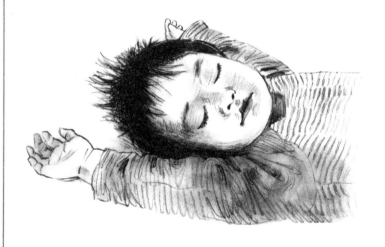

FUN FACT

At three months, babies' sleep starts to look more like that of an adult, with four distinct stages, known as nREM1, nREM2, nREM3 and REM. But their sleep cycles are much shorter than an adult's, lasting around forty minutes, compared to the ninety minutes of an adult sleep cycle.

PARENTING Q&A

Q. *Do all babies experience a four-month sleep regression?*

A. *Absolutely not! Each baby has a unique sleep pattern, and while four months is a common time for parents to struggle with sleep, many sail through this period with no sleep difficulties at all.*

is possible that this can cause some babies to become more fractious in their sleep. In addition, this is often the age of increased motor skills (such as rolling), which can also impact sleep. Four months is also a bit of a milestone in baby sleep, as it is the bridge between immature newborn sleep and more mature adult-like sleep in terms of a change in sleep cycles and sleep consolidation. Don't worry if your baby's sleep does seem to get worse at this age; it is not a sign that you have done anything wrong or need to change anything. The more disturbed sleep won't last for ever.

At this age, most babies are napping either three or four times per day, with each nap lasting around thirty to sixty minutes. Total sleep over a twenty-four-hour period is usually around fourteen hours.

Sleep at five to six months

By the time your baby is six months old, they will sleep for about thirteen hours in a twenty-four-hour period. They will likely take three naps per day, with each lasting around thirty to sixty minutes, although it is not unusual for babies to nap less – or more – than this. Remember, every baby is unique.

Night waking is still usual in five- to six-month-olds, with only 16 per cent regularly sleeping through the night. Most babies of this age wake three times each night (a slight increase from three months of age), which often confuses parents. However, this is such a busy period of development, and sleep can often be unpredictable due to these neurological and physical changes.

By six months, the differentiation of a baby's sleep into four distinct stages has fully transitioned and their sleep looks much more like that of an adult. Their sleep cycles are still roughly only fifty minutes long, though – a little over half the length of an adult's.

Schedules vs routines

At this stage, you may find people recommending that you get your baby onto a schedule to try to improve their sleep. The idea of feeding a baby based on the clock and trying to get them to nap and go to sleep at night according to a timetable is outdated, but one that still persists. Strict feeding and nap

---

PARENTING Q&A

Q. *Will weaning my five-month-old onto solids help her sleep? It has been very unpredictable lately and I wonder if she's waking so much because she's hungry?*

A. *Probably not, I'm afraid. This is a common age for baby sleep to become unpredictable, with more night wakes occurring than in the previous months. Research has shown that the timing of introducing solid foods makes no difference to babies' sleep as they grow.*[10]

Anthropology Titbit In hunter-gatherer societies, such as the !Kung, who live on the edge of the Kalahari desert, babies spend most of the day and night being held and are rarely put down. The Beng people, in the Côte d'Ivoire, carry their babies on their backs in carriers as they work. Both societies consider holding and carrying a baby a good way to get them to sleep.

schedules don't improve baby sleep in the long term, but can be stressful to implement.

Following a routine, however, whereby you do the same things in the same order to introduce some predictability, can really help sleep. Don't worry about clockwatching, though – this is more about what you do than when you do it.

Here is an example of a bedtime routine you might follow at this age:

- A little quiet playtime in your living area (just five or ten minutes is enough)
- Bath time, or just a wipe down and nappy change
- A little massage in the bedroom, with some soft music playing
- Changing into a fresh Babygro and sleep sac, if you use one
- Breast- or bottle-feed
- Cuddles until they fall asleep

There's no feeling like the feeling of holding your world in your arms.
Unknown

Contact naps – AKA why your baby only naps when you hold them

Many parents worry that their baby only seems happy to nap when they are holding them, waking as soon as they put them down. There is good reason for this. Contact naps, as I call them, help babies to feel safe. The warmth of your skin and the reassuring beating of your heart helps them to feel connected to you and reminds them of life in utero.

Humans are carry mammals, meaning that our babies are designed to nap in our arms, just like those of other carry mammals (including apes, and marsupials such as kangaroos). Contact naps are a great way of forcing you to take a break, too, and rest while your baby sleeps. If you do want to get on with some work, then a good, supportive baby carrier or sling allows you to have your hands free, while your baby gets the close contact they need to nap well.

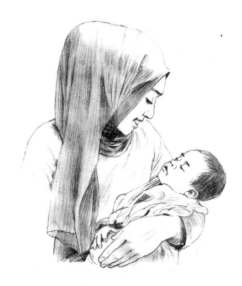

This is also a nice age to introduce a bedtime story, if you haven't already done so. You could read this during your baby's milk feed, or during cuddles afterwards, if they are still awake. Or you could read a story as part of the quiet playtime at the start of the routine above.

Social and psychological development from three to six months

The three-to-six-month period is a wonderful time for social development. Your baby is so much more interested in the world and interacting with others, and their personality really starts to shine through.

You will probably notice that your baby has much more awareness of where they are during these months, and they are able to discern when they are in a new environment. Some babies may become unsettled when they find themselves somewhere new or surrounded by people they don't know at this age. If this happens, they are likely to require more reassurance from you, which usually takes the shape of needing to be in your arms. Sometimes people refer to babies who cry if they are not being held by their parents as 'clingy', but this is a normal, healthy reaction, indicating that you make them

Parent Observation 'We found that skin-to-skin contact still worked really well to calm our son when he was struggling with (what we think was) teething pain when he was five months old. He was always so much calmer if we stripped off and cuddled together under a warm blanket or went in the bath with him.'

> *FUN FACT*
> *When a baby is three months of age, social synchrony*
> *(a strong attachment, whereby parent and baby react to each*
> *other's emotions and actions) can predict how well they will*
> *interact with their peers when they are older.*[11]

feel safe in an unknown environment. Remember, everything is new to a baby.

Unsurprisingly, your baby thrives on familiarity at this age, enjoying predictability, such as repeated routines and actions (the same song sung time and again, for instance), especially if they involve you. Their bond with you is the driver for all their future relationships, and the best way to grow this is to respond to your baby – pick them up, touch them, play with them, sing to them, talk to them and never, ever be afraid of being too loving or too nurturing. It is not possible to spoil a baby with cuddles.

Language and communication from three to six months

At the start of this period, your baby will likely be making cooing, grunting and squealing sounds. By the end, however, they have made quite a jump in their language development and their babbling will start to take on more language-type sounds, such as repeating a letter sound. By four months of age, babies can also recognise the difference between the five vowel sounds when they are spoken.[12] This all develops organically, as your baby watches you and listens to everything you say. You will notice them increasingly turning towards noises

> *FUN FACT*
> *By four months of age, most babies will appreciate humour,*
> *and you will likely notice their first laugh during this period.*[13]

and looking at you when you speak as they become more and more interested in language.

How to help language development

- Read to your baby as often as you can.

- Speak to your baby regularly. For instance, you could narrate your day, telling them what you are doing.

- Copy their noises.

- Pause and listen when they make a noise and respond, mimicking a conversation.

- Use their name.

- Sing nursery rhymes.

- Adults/carers should refer to themselves as Mummy/Daddy/Grandma/Grandad, as applicable.

- Look at them when you talk and make sure they can see your whole face as much as possible.

> It's way too early for him to be talking anyhow, but I see in his eyes something, and I see in his eyes a voice and I see in his eyes a whole new set of words.
> *Sherman Alexie, American novelist*

Play ideas for babies from three to six months

You are still the main source of entertainment for your baby – your movements, words and everyday interaction with them are more stimulating than you could ever imagine. As mentioned above, they will start to appreciate humour at this age, so funny faces, blowing raspberries and the like will usually be well received.

A good focus at this age, if you want to incorporate specific play ideas, are toys that help to encourage your baby's physical development (such as tummy-time mats) and exploration of objects through touch, sight and sound. Special rings or cushions to support them while they sit for short periods of time are also useful.

Recommended toys

- **A rattle** or similar noise-making object – move this around in front of your baby's face to attract their attention and gaze, encouraging them to grasp and move it to make a noise. This will help their hand–eye co-ordination.

- **Balls** – a brightly coloured soft ball with a bell inside or a sensory ball (usually made with rubber and different textures), small enough for them to grasp and move from hand to hand will, again, improve their co-ordination and the noise will help to hold their attention.

- **A baby gym**, for them to lie underneath: this allows them to reach out and try to grab objects, or bat them to make a noise.

PARENTING Q&A

Q. *I've read that tickling babies isn't good for them. Is this true?*

A. *Tickling can be very overwhelming for babies. It's highly sensory and, unlike adults, they are unable to ask you to stop or to move away when they have had enough. It's therefore better to avoid deliberate tickling until your little one is much older.*

- **Toys with large buttons** that they can press to make something pop up, light up or make a noise. It doesn't need to have a variety of different buttons and functions – remember, babies of this age like repeating actions, so two or three different buttons is plenty for them.

- **A teething ring or toy** – something that has been specially designed to be chewed and has different sensory textures for the baby to feel with their gums.

- **Fabric baby books,** featuring bold colours and illustrations, for them to learn how to pick up and hold a page. Choose ones that are able to withstand chewing!

A quick note: do remember that babies tend to put everything in their mouths at this age, so do ensure that any toy your baby has is safe.

Your baby has changed rapidly during this period, in both body and mind, and every week they seem to have developed a new skill. As they move into the next three months, you will see even more rapid development, with perhaps their first word and the new-found skill of mobility! Chapter 4 covers all this and more, as we learn how your six- to nine-month-old will develop.

4

Six to Nine Months

Congratulations on your baby's half birthday! By now, you're probably feeling more confident as a parent, and likely finding it much easier to understand their cues and needs. Months six to nine bring about even more change, the major developments being summed up with one word: mobility. But your baby's new-found movement skills are by no means the only thing going on – there's lots more that just isn't visible yet.

How the brain develops from six to nine months

At this age, the brain is still very much focused on growing new synaptic connections, with an emphasis still on the cerebellum (the part responsible for movement and balance) and the hippocampus (responsible for memory and learning). The more learning is reinforced at this age, the more likely the

> I think that I see something deeper, more infinite, more eternal than the ocean in the expression of the eyes of a little baby when it wakes in the morning and coos or laughs because it sees the sun shining in its cradle.
> *Vincent van Gogh, artist*

baby is to retain the skill as they grow. Research has found that by the time they are six months old, babies are able to tell the difference between photographs of two different human faces.[1] Surprisingly, they are also able to tell the difference between photographs of two difference monkey faces, something most adults are incapable of. If the babies are repeatedly assessed for their monkey-differentiating abilities, they retain the skill until at least nine months of age; however, without repeated testing, they quickly lose it – just like adults. Practically speaking, for parents and carers this means that rather than viewing repeated activities and behaviours as boring and unstimulating for our babies, we should understand that they are key to reinforcing learning.

By seven months, your baby's brain is busy preparing for their first conversations, even though it may be several more months before they speak their first words. Research has found that their brains are active in a part of the brain known as 'Broca's area',[2] found in the frontal lobe and responsible for speech-related activities, including the motor movements of the tongue and lips and the regulation of breathing during speaking. The activity in this part of the brain, before a baby can actually speak, indicates that their brain is busy preparing for speech by first analysing the motions needed as a result of experience and observation.

A study looking at the impact of language on the brain of seven-month-old babies found that they were more responsive, with more activity in the frontal cortex of the brain,

Neuroscience Nugget By the time a baby is eight months old, they will have around five hundred trillion connections between neurons in their brain.

Neuroscience Nugget A baby's growing brain uses up around 60 per cent of their total metabolic energy each day. An adult brain, in contrast, uses closer to 25 per cent.

when parents spoke in high-pitched tones and sounded happy.[3] (This style of joyful babytalk is often referred to as 'motherese' or 'parentese', and is usually adopted entirely unconsciously by adults when they are around babies.) Using a technique known as near-infrared spectroscopy (NIRS), researchers studied the levels of oxygen in different areas of a baby's brain, while the babies sat on their parents' laps and were spoken to. Fascinatingly now, we have the technology to prove that babies' brains thrive on this type of communication that parents have been naturally using for centuries.

Research with seven-month-old babies has shown that their somatosensory cortex (a part of the brain which runs over the top of the head, from ear to ear, and is responsible for sensations including touch) is developing rapidly at this stage.[4] This part of the brain activates when babies are gently touched on their hands and their feet, and also when they observe somebody else being touched, but feel no touch themselves. This recognition of the experience of touch – i.e. whether they or someone else is being touched – helps babies

Parent Observation 'When my son was six months old, he used to love me stroking his hands and feet. I used to sing "This little piggy" as I stroked his fingers and toes, and he would beam a huge smile at me. It's such a lovely memory now.'

to understand and imitate what they see their parents and carers doing, ultimately becoming an early precursor to developing a sense of empathy for others.

Physical development from six to nine months

Months six through nine are all about your baby's increasing mobility skills. If you haven't done so already, now is definitely the time to think about introducing some babyproofing safety measures into your home.

Physical milestones

Your baby will likely be rapidly gaining physical skills now, enabling them to engage fully with the world around them and speeding their learning.

Six to seven months

By the time they turn seven months, your baby may be able to sit without support and will probably use their arms to steady themselves. When they are supported in a standing position, they will bear most of their weight on their legs and will enjoy bending their knees in a bouncing motion. You will probably notice a difference in the way they reach for, pick up and hold toys at this age, as their movements become more accurate.

FUN FACT
Although they will soon be crawling, babies don't yet have kneecaps. Their patellas won't begin to fuse and ossify (turn from cartilage to bone) until after their second birthdays.

Keeping your mobile baby safe

The best way to babyproof your home is to get onto the floor, in a crawling position, and look at each room from the angle of your baby. What can you see that might present a hazard? The following are recommended:

- Make sure any dangling cords are removed or fixed safely out of reach – for instance those on roller blinds, or electrical cords.
- Fix freestanding pieces of furniture, such as chests of drawers, to the wall, to ensure your baby can't pull them onto themselves.
- Move fragile objects, particularly those made from glass or ceramic, well out of reach.
- Move cleaning products out of reach, or use cupboard locks to ensure your baby cannot get hold of them.
- Look for sharp edges, such as those on coffee tables, and consider changing pieces of furniture, or using corner protectors.
- Check for hot pipes, leading to radiators and consider using pipe covering to protect little hands from burns.
- Invest in a fireguard, if you have an open fire.

Note: one common piece of safety proofing that you don't need if you live in the UK is electrical socket covers. All UK power sockets have internal shutters installed in them to prevent children from getting electric shocks. Unfortunately, there are no safety regulations for socket covers and well-meaning parents may inadvertently make a safe socket *unsafe* by installing them.

Anthropology Titbit In some areas of Bali, when babies are almost seven months old, a ceremony known as '*nyabutan*' is conducted to mark their birthday by the Wuku calendar (a Balinese calendar with 210 days per year). Offerings are made to the spirits to remove any negativity that the baby may have come into contact with.

They use something called a 'raking grasp' to pick things up, moving all their fingers in a raking motion to get hold of something (a little like a claw machine you find at an amusement arcade – see illustration below).

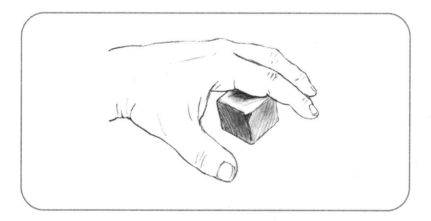

Visually speaking, by six months, babies can perceive depth in pictures, as well as in real life.[5] Their vision is much more mature and they can see across a room.

Seven to eight months

At this age, your baby will become more skilled at passing objects, particularly smaller ones, from one hand to the other. They will also likely progress to something called an 'inferior pincer grasp' (below left) to pick up small items. This involves using the pads of their thumb and index finger and is the first step towards using a full pincer grasp (below right), which uses the tips of both the thumb and index finger and is more precise).

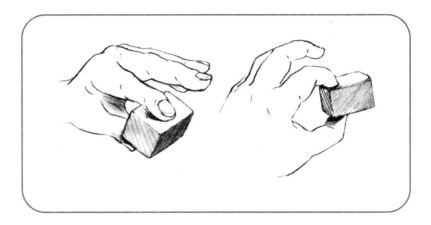

Your baby will still be working towards crawling at this age, and you will probably notice they spend more time on their hands and knees and practise rocking backwards and forwards a lot. In fact, 50 per cent of babies start to crawl by eight months of age.

Neuroscience Nugget The neurons responsible for vision in a baby's brain speed up their message sending from around three months of age. This signalling peaks in intensity by the time a baby reaches eight months of age, correlating with them being intensely interested in the world around them.

Eight to nine months

Your baby stands a good chance of learning to crawl by the end of this month. (Although not all babies crawl – it's estimated that 10 per cent skip this stage entirely.)

They work hard on their grasp, too, during this month and will likely have mastered the pincer grasp by the time they turn nine months. They will probably be able to watch a moving object and reach out and grab it. You may also notice that they learn to clap during this period, too.

Research conducted in the 1960s found that when babies learn to crawl, they already have a good level of depth perception.[6] The 'visual cliff' experiment set up a sheet of Plexiglass over a shallow platform at one end and a deeper one at the other (see below). The surfaces were all covered in

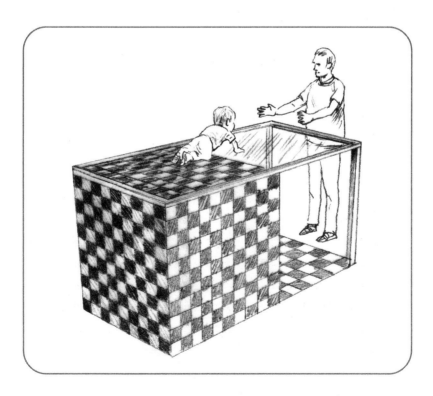

Anthropology Titbit The babies of the Au people of Papua New Guinea don't crawl because they are carried almost constantly until they begin walking.

a checkerboard pattern. Babies aged between six and fourteen months of age were placed on the shallow platform and their parent or carer waited on the other deeper side and called them over. The experiment found that 92 per cent of babies refused to crawl to their carer over the 'deep' end, even though there was Plexiglass covering it, indicating that by the time they crawl, babies already have well-developed depth perception.

PARENTING Q&A

Q. *My baby shuffles along the floor on his bum and shows no interest in crawling. Is this OK?*

A. *Bum shuffling is a variation of normal development, and if they get around quickly in this way, there isn't much motivation for babies to learn to crawl. Bum shufflers are often a little late to walk, but there is no problem with the bum shuffling itself. If you would like to encourage your baby's walking development, you could work on helping your baby to build core strength, which in turn will help them to balance as they learn to take their first steps. You can help your baby's core strength by encouraging them to stand against you, using you as a support, and by building more tummy time into their day. Both of these are great for your baby's core muscle development.*

Babies love dancing

Babies seem to be born with a predisposition to move to the beat of music. Research has found that babies under one year can dance in time with music, moving their limbs and torso in a rhythmical manner.[7] Babies of this age seem to focus on the rhythm of the music more than any other aspect (such as melodies or voices). As well as being able to keep in time, babies are more likely to smile when dancing to the beat!

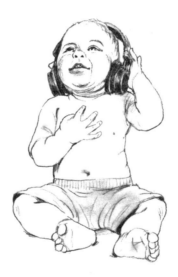

Parent Observation 'Whenever I had a particularly bad day with my baby daughter, I would put on the soundtrack to *The Lion King* and dance around the room with her in a baby carrier. She would always be so much happier and more relaxed, and it really helped to lighten my mood, too.'

Feeding and eating from six to nine months

Six to nine months is possibly the most exciting time in your baby's life so far when it comes to eating, because they are now ready for solid foods. Despite what the word 'weaning' suggests, however, it doesn't mean that they are ready to leave milk feeds behind; milk forms an important part of their diet for many months yet. The introduction of solid food is complementary to milk.

Signs that your baby is ready for solids

So far in this book, we have focused on signs that are commonly misinterpreted as weaning readiness, but the following are the real indications:

- They are around six months old.
- They can sit up unaided (with a little support if necessary).
- They have good head control and neck strength.
- They have lost their 'tongue-thrust reflex' (when their tongue instantly pokes any food away that enters their mouth) and can swallow foods.
- They can co-ordinate their hands, eyes and mouth, by looking at food, grabbing it, putting it in their mouth and chewing and swallowing it.

Don't worry if your baby doesn't have any teeth yet, they can still eat solid foods perfectly well by mushing the food with their gums.

PARENTING Q&A

Q. *My baby still needs a cushion behind her to support her while she sits. Does this mean she's not ready to wean?*

A. *No, this is fine. Your baby doesn't have to sit completely unaided; she just needs to have good head control and be able to sit upright, even if she needs a cushion to help her stay that way.*

The difference between gagging and choking

However you choose to wean your baby, it is important to understand the signs of choking, and how they differ from gagging.

Choking	Gagging
A medical emergency in which food is partially, or fully, blocking the windpipe	A normal physiological response to something touching the back of the throat.
Often silent, or an ineffective coughing	Usually very noisy, with loud retching sounds
Face may be pale or blue and lips begin to turn blue	Face usually shows some reddening
Nothing is brought up	Often accompanied by spitting food or vomiting
Baby needs immediate help	Baby will resolve independently

Many parents and carers are alarmed by gagging because it sounds scary, but it is normal and common. It is not an indication that your baby is not ready for solids.

Note: if you haven't already done so, now is a good time to take an infant first-aid class – preferably one that covers how to manage choking and infant CPR.

Parent Observation 'I ate a lot of spicy food during my pregnancy and my baby laps up strong flavours now. It's so funny to see that he loves what I used to eat during pregnancy!'

Baby-led vs traditional weaning

There are two main approaches to weaning: baby-led and traditional. Baby-led weaning involves giving your baby finger-sized pieces of food and preloaded spoons, allowing them to feed themselves from the very start. Traditional weaning involves making purées and feeding them with a spoon (and later introducing finger foods). The key difference between the two is autonomy. In traditional weaning, the process is very much led by the parent or carer and the baby takes a more passive role. In baby-led weaning, the baby is in control of their eating experience from the start, with the parent or carer assuming the more passive role. Many hypothesise that this autonomy makes baby-led weaning a more positive approach for the baby, and could lead to a better relationship with eating as they grow.

A guide to recommended first foods – and what to avoid

The foods that you offer your baby during weaning can impact their relationship with food for years to come. We have learned in previous chapters that babies favour sugary and salty tastes, and it can be tempting, especially with sugar, to feed them lots of sweet foods (such as fruit purées) when you are weaning, as they are usually well received. But a better approach is to stick with savoury tastes – in particular vegetables – to avoid even more of a preference for sweet foods.

Recommended first foods	Foods to avoid
Green vegetables, such as broccoli, spinach and green beans	Honey (can contain bacteria which can cause botulism)
Root vegetables, such as carrots, swede and sweet potatoes	Ready-made baby snacks (can contain a lot of added sugar and salt)
Other vegetables, such as butternut squash and more savoury fruit, such as avocado	Baby rice (has little nutritional value and carries a risk of arsenic poisoning)
Eggs and full-fat dairy, such as unsweetened yoghurt	Sweetened yoghurts and fromage frais
Fish and meat without bones	Higher-salt foods, such as those made with ready-made stock cubes and gravy

How should you start to offer solids?

When you start weaning, it's always a good idea to offer solid food after a milk feed. Remember, the solid food isn't meant to replace their milk, but rather be complementary to it, so you don't want to fill them up on solids which, at this stage, will likely contain far fewer nutrients than their milk. As they get older and start to eat more, you can offer solid food before milk, but for the first three months at least, it is usually better to focus on milk feeds first.

Pick a time when your baby is naturally calm and happy – for instance, when they have recently woken from a nap and aren't tired. Go at their pace and don't try to make them eat more than they are interested in or to persuade them to continue eating something they don't like. Finally, expect lots of mess! Mess is important when your baby is learning to eat solids because it adds to the sensory experience. Don't be tempted to rush in and clean them up too soon, instead allowing them to explore the food fully with their hands.

PARENTING Q&A

Q. *We started weaning a couple of weeks ago, and our baby isn't really interested in food. Most of it ends up on his bib or highchair. Is this OK?*

A. *Yes! Parents tend to have a romanticised picture of what weaning will look like, with happy, smiling babies eating whatever they are offered. In reality, though, a lot of the food will be spat out, ending up on the floor, on the baby and on you, with little being digested. This is fine, because the first tastes of food are more about learning and exploring and less about nutrition.*

Sleep development from six to nine months

Many sources of parenting information imply that most babies sleep through the night by six months of age. Unfortunately, this commonly held belief is incorrect. While some may be sleeping quite soundly during this period, many will still be waking and feeding regularly throughout the night. The period between six and nine months is incredibly changeable sleep-wise. Let's look at what you can expect:

Sleep at six to seven months

Six-month-olds sleep for an average of ten and a half hours at night and an average of three hours in the daytime. Daytime sleep is usually split between three naps, each lasting for around an hour each, although it isn't uncommon for there to be one longer nap and two shorter ones. Research has found that 50 per cent of six-month-olds are still waking regularly at

FUN FACT
When sleeping through the night doesn't mean sleeping all night!: when you read recommendations for the total hours of sleep a baby should have at night, what you are not told is that these totals are calculated according to the time of bedtime and the time of waking in the morning.
They don't subtract any time the baby may have been awake in the night for feeds and cuddles. So, for instance, if a six-month-old goes to sleep at 7.30 p.m. and wakes at 6 a.m., they would be considered to have had ten and a half hours of sleep, even if they woke up every hour throughout the night.

night, but it varies a lot between babies – so it's important not to compare your baby's sleep to others of the same age.[8]

A lot of parents expect sleep to improve once babies start eating solid food, but weaning often makes them wake more. This is because the change can initially be a little unsettling for them; there may be a chance of allergies and gastrointestinal discomfort; and if they are taking less milk in the daytime due to eating more solids, they often want more milk at night.

One positive improvement that occurs at this age is that the time it takes to get babies to sleep usually reduces. Research indicates that the average six-month-old takes around twenty minutes to fall asleep.[9]

Sleep at seven to eight months

Sleep between seven and eight months is often slightly easier. Weaning is no longer brand new and the sleep changes that may have occurred because of it often settle down again. Night waking is still common, though. Babies of this age still sleep for an average of around ten and a half hours at night, but, remember, that's from bedtime to morning wake time, regardless of night wakes. Naps can often drop down to two per day. Initially, when your baby drops a nap, their usual rhythms may be disrupted and sleep may be a little erratic for a few weeks; however, a new pattern has usually emerged by the end of this period.

Anthropology Titbit In Bali, babies spend the evening with their parents and participate in celebrations and rituals at night. Sometimes they fall asleep in their parents' arms, sometimes they stay awake – either is considered to be fine.

> *FUN FACT*
>
> *When scientists research infant sleep and use the term 'sleep through the night', they usually mean a period of not waking for five to six hours. Most parents, however, define 'sleeping through the night' as the baby going to sleep at bedtime and not waking until the morning. The next time you read about a piece of research that mentions babies 'sleeping through the night', remember they probably aren't talking about sleeping the whole night through.*

This is a common age for parents to move their baby into their own room. SIDS (cot death) guidelines state that your baby should be in the same room as you for all sleep (day and night) for at least the first six months. That doesn't mean you should rush to move them into their own room the day they turn seven months, though. Some parents do find that their babies sleep better in their own sleep space, while others find that they wake more and that settling them takes more time and effort because they have to get up and go to a different room each time. Don't feel pressured to move your baby into their own room if you are not ready.

Sleep at eight to nine months

Babies of this age still sleep for an average of around ten and a half hours each night, but their daytime naps have now reduced to a total of between two and two and a half hours. Most babies of this age still nap twice per day, with each nap lasting around an hour. Again, it is not unusual for one nap to be slightly longer than the other, for instance, one lasting for an hour and the other lasting for an hour and a half.

Is sleep training effective?

Many parents consider sleep training at some point in their baby's first year. The lure of adverts promising undisturbed nights and better development for your baby is strong – but is sleep training really effective?

While sleep-training techniques can work in the sense that they can teach babies to be quiet at night and not to cry out to their parents, what they don't do is to make the baby sleep more (as opposed to being awake but not crying) or have any long-term positive effects on their sleep. Sleep is a question of development – neurological and physical – and emotional maturity. Sadly, there are no short cuts here, and trying to get a baby to sleep through the night before these things have been established is about as effective as trying to teach them to ride a bike before they can walk.

PARENTING Q&A

Q. *My seven-month-old seems to be dropping down to two naps per day. Previously he napped at about 9 a.m., 12.30 p.m. and 4 p.m. What sort of times should we be looking at for the two naps he seems to want now?*

A. *When babies drop to two naps, it's usually the midday one that disappears, and you will probably find that making the first nap a little later and the second a little earlier will work better when he is on two. Aiming for around 10 a.m. and 2 or 3 p.m. often works well.*

Baby sleep can often become less predictable again at the nine-month mark – something we will look at more in the next chapter. Research has found that 40 per cent of parents are concerned about their babies' difficult sleep at this age.[10] The good news is that the apparent regression in sleep isn't permanent, and it isn't a sign that you have done something wrong – it's normal and it will pass naturally, given time.

Social and psychological development from six to nine months

Between six and nine months, your baby's emotions are developing rapidly. When they were younger, these centred only on two extremes of stress and calmness, but now they also include fear, sadness, happiness and anger.

Your baby will likely become increasingly wary around strangers during these months and may be upset if somebody they don't know talks to them or tries to pick them up. This isn't an indication that you have done something wrong to make them shy or antisocial. Far from it – this wariness of strangers shows that they feel safe with you and that they just need more time to learn to feel safe and secure with others.

Your baby is always watching and observing you, and although you may be worried that you are sometimes boring

> You inspire them to be kinder, better, greater, more successful, more impactful. Perhaps it's the new-found clarity I have as a father knowing that my son will always be watching what I do, mimicking my behaviour.
> *Prince Harry*

and wonder if they need more entertainment or time with others to teach them social skills, they actually learn everything they need from their daily interactions with you. Whenever you speak to them, react to their movements or noises, hold them, read to them and look at them, you are teaching them how to interact with others and how to socialise.

Research looking at seven-month-old babies has found that they observe much more than we think they do, especially when it comes to following our actions and choices.[11] Scientists asked adults to select from two different toys, while the babies observed. The babies were then presented with the same two toys. When they selected the same toy as the adult they had previously observed, activity in the part of the brain responsible for motor control was heightened, indicating that the babies understood the adult's moves and were able to consciously copy them. This research highlights that babies in this age group are already developing conscious social behaviour, based upon mirroring the actions of the adults around them.

Scientists have also discovered that babies as young as six months are developing morals. Researchers acted out a puppet show for babies between six and ten months, demonstrating some characters helping others, and others not engaging in any helping.[12] At the end of the show, babies were allowed to select one of the characters they had just seen. In 80 per cent of cases, the babies selected the altruistic (the helper) characters. Another aspect of the experiment saw researchers acting out

> Children are human beings to whom respect is due,
> superior to us by reason of their innocence and of
> the greater possibilities of their future.
> *Maria Montessori, educator*

The Tronick 'still face' experiment

In 1975, Edward Tronick, a psychologist from Boston, USA, observed parent-and-infant pairs in two different scenarios. In the first, he instructed the parent to fully engage with the baby – to smile, talk and interact with them as usual. In the second scenario, the parent was to adopt a 'still face', showing no emotion at all and no interaction. When the parent was engaging, the babies were happy and smiling and fully engaged with them. In the still-face scenario, the babies tried repeatedly to get the parents to interact with them as usual, and when the parents remained detached, the babies quickly became withdrawn and distressed, looking away from them. This experiment shows how reliant babies are on their parents and carers to interact with them. Babies are wired for connection with us and struggle emotionally if they do not receive it.

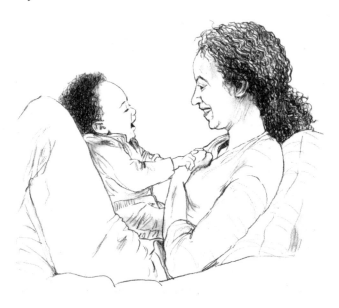

a different puppet show – this time with a helpful character, as well as one who stole something from another. At the end of the show, the babies were encouraged to choose one of the characters and, again, the majority selected the helpful character. They were also prompted to take a treat from one of the characters. The majority chose the character they'd seen stealing, indicating a belief that it was better to take from someone who had stolen than from someone who had been helpful.

Language and communication from six to nine months

Although your baby hasn't yet spoken their first word, their language skills are rapidly developing. Before they turn six months old, they may recognise words that are familiar to them, but they don't understand their meaning. Understanding, as well as recognition of words, however, starts to develop during the six-to-nine-month period. You can expect your baby to begin to understand certain words you use frequently, such as 'food', 'bath' and 'toy'.

Your baby will also be busy practising their conversational skills, and you will likely notice that they reply to you and pause while you speak, indicating that they understand the

FUN FACT
It is common for parents to believe that their baby is saying 'dada' as their first word, but 'd' is a sound that babies often make at this age and 'd, d' can easily be interpreted as 'dada'. Interestingly, 'mama', or 'm, m' is a harder sound for them to produce, hence it usually appears after 'd, d'.

Parent Observation 'I must have sung "Wind the bobbin up" about a thousand times between six and twelve months. My son absolutely loved it, especially when we did the actions together. When we did the clapping hands he would shriek with laughter.'

social exchange that happens during a conversation. At this point, they will practise making the sounds of consonants and will often string several together – for instance, 'b,b,b,b' or 'd, d, d, d'.

You will probably find that your baby is more vocal when it comes to indicating their emotions now and they are likely to make different noises depending on how they are feeling. Once you learn their noises, it can often make taking care of them easier, as you are able to understand how they feel and meet their needs better.

Finally, you will find that your baby not only recognises their own name at this age, but actively responds to it, smiling when you use it and looking around the room if somebody else calls them by their name.

Play ideas for babies from six to nine months

You are still the primary source of entertainment for your baby at this age. They love to laugh when you make silly faces and noises, or when you dance with them, and they are becoming more interested in books when you read together. Babies learn by repetition, and you will notice this in their play. For instance, when they drop a toy and you pick it up, they will drop it again (and again and again). This repeated dropping is not only a great source of entertainment, but also means they are learning about gravity and learning to trust you to help them every time you pick the toy up again. Don't be afraid of repetition in play and entertainment – you may worry that your baby is bored with you singing the same nursery rhyme over and over, but they love it, and get as much (if not more) from you singing it for the hundredth time as they did the first time.

Recommended toys

The best toys for six- to nine-month-olds focus on their growing interest in manipulating the world around them and their increasing manual dexterity, as they develop their pincer grip:

- **A set of plastic stacking cups** (which can double as great pouring toys in the bath as they get older)

- **Wooden building blocks** that they can bang together or stack in ever-bigger towers

- **Toy drums** – or any toy that can be banged

- **Toys with buttons** they can press to create a sound or lids that they can press down to close

- **Board books** (ones that can withstand banging and chewing), especially those with pictures of everyday objects to help broaden their vocabulary and where they can – eventually – point to pictures of the words as you say them

- **Vinyl bath books**, to chew and practise turning the pages at bath time

As well as specific toys, babies are incredibly interested in everyday objects at this age. Don't underestimate the value

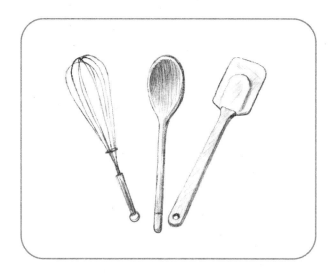

of playing with a simple kitchen whisk, an old purse or wallet or handbag, a wooden spoon (used to hit things!) and some interesting textured fabric. Many people like to gather up interesting, baby-friendly, everyday objects and keep them together in a 'treasure basket'. Treasure baskets can entertain babies for far longer than many baby toys, which tend to have limited play potential – the other bonus being that you will often already have the items lying around your house, so no extra expense is needed.

Six to nine months is such a lovely period of development, with so many firsts – not least your baby's first taste of solid foods and the first time they become truly mobile. Social interactions and humour are really developing during this time, too, and you are often rewarded with conversations and belly laughs. Of course, the firsts don't end here, with so much more to come over the next few months. We will look at some of the milestones you can expect to see before their first birthday in the next chapter.

5

Nine to Twelve Months

Levels of both physical and psychological development in the last three months of your baby's first year are astounding. By the end of this period, they will be well on the way to walking and talking, making great strides socially, too. Let's take a look at some of the major milestones at this stage and what to expect as they approach the end of their first year.

How the brain develops from nine to twelve months

Forming new synaptic connections and myelinating pre-existing ones to speed messages between the brain's neurons, as described on page 9, is the focus of brain development at this time.

During this period, the corpus callosum (the part of the brain containing bundles of nerve fibres that sits between both hemispheres, connecting them) is expanding in size. This enables your baby's brain to send messages between both sides of the brain more effectively. Also, deep in the brain, the limbic system – comprising the hypothalamus, thalamus,

Neuroscience Nugget Between months nine and twelve, a baby's brain grows by 0.5 per cent every day.

amygdala and hippocampus (among others) – is rapidly developing at this point.

The limbic system is responsible for behavioural and emotional instinctive responses, especially those linked to survival (such as fear and the fight-or-flight stress response) and habitual and reward-seeking behaviours. This part of the brain also plays a strong role in memories and how they impact our feelings. The development of the limbic system means that your baby will be increasingly feeling big emotions. Perhaps the strongest indication of this stage of development is the emergence of separation anxiety; when babies with a strong attachment to their parents and caregivers feel scared when they are separated from them. (We will talk about separation anxiety much more later in this chapter.) Research has found that the more parents nurture and respond to their babies at this age, the greater the size of their limbic system in later childhood.[1]

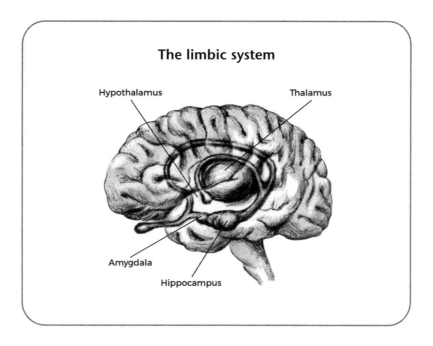

The limbic system

Hypothalamus

Thalamus

Amygdala

Hippocampus

Neuroscience Nugget   Grey and white matter in the brain is so called because the absence or presence of myelin causes brain tissue to change colour (myelin is composed of around 70 per cent lipids, or fats). Areas with high levels of myelination are whiter, whereas those with less are seen as grey.

When do babies form memories?

Your nine- to twelve-month-old's memory function will take several more years to fully develop and become the type of memory we know as adults. Despite this, babies do have a degree of memory; if they didn't, it would be impossible for them to learn and grow cognitively and to develop physical skills. Research has found that something known as implicit memory (memories that are acquired and used unconsciously) is stable in nine-month-olds,[2] whereas explicit memory (memories that can be consciously recalled at will) begins to develop between eight and ten months, and is associated with significant growth in the hippocampus.

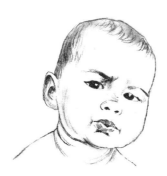

Implicit memories are the mainstay during infancy, with explicit memories in the minority until the child is of school age. This explains why, as adults, we struggle to remember anything that happened before the age of two and a half.[3]

Myelination continues throughout this period, still with a strong focus on parts of the brain responsible for movement and sensory experiences. Myelination in areas of the brain responsible for higher cognitive functions is still a long way from completion.

Although it may seem that your baby acquires new skills overnight at this age, research indicates that the learning behind them happens constantly and consistently.[4] For instance, it may seem as if they have become vocal very suddenly, and it can be tempting to view this as a 'leap', arising from quickly acquired skills. However, it is the result of an accumulation of many months of largely unnoticed physical, social and linguistic development.

Physical development from nine to twelve months

The milestones your baby achieves during months nine to twelve are divided into two main types: gross and fine motor skills. Gross motor skills refer to those that use the body's large muscles to produce a big movement, such as moving the legs when learning to walk. Fine motor skills refer to those that use small muscles (or muscle groups) for smaller, more refined movements, such as using the fingers to pick up an object. Fine motor skills are all about dexterity, whereas gross motor skills are all about strength.

> When a child is learning to walk and falls down
> fifty times, they never think to themselves,
> 'Maybe this isn't for me.'
> *Unknown*

Physical milestones

Your baby's whole body is hard at work during this period, focusing on acquiring more mobility and fine motor skills. Let's look at what you can expect over the next three months.

Nine to ten months

Most babies will have mastered crawling by the time they are ten months and will usually start to pull themselves up on a piece of solid furniture. Although they often master pulling themselves up at this age, it takes a few weeks until they are able to get themselves back down again; until then, they will probably need your help. By the end of this period, your baby will probably be able to sit themselves up from lying on their stomach. They may start to point to items they want or poke things they are interested in, and they will track with their eyes objects that fall from a higher surface. At this age, they will be working on their pincer grip, grasping smaller objects with the tips of their thumbs and index fingers.

PARENTING Q&A

Q. *When should I buy my baby their first pair of shoes?*

A. *It may be tempting to rush out and buy your baby their first pair of shoes as soon as they start to cruise or take their first steps. Try to resist the urge, though, as it's much better for them to remain barefoot for now. If you are worried about their feet getting cold or dirty, then look at soft soled or so-called 'barefoot shoes', designed specifically for developing feet.*

Ten to eleven months

Ten-month-olds can now squat back down to the floor after they have pulled themselves up and many will be able to stand unassisted. Once your baby has mastered standing (and sitting again) they will usually quickly progress to cruising – moving around with a shuffling-foot motion while holding on to pieces of furniture. Cruising is the last gross motor skill they need before they learn how to walk. By the end of this period, they may have learned how to wave, especially when saying 'bye bye' to somebody.

Eleven to twelve months

This is an exciting age, as it will often involve your baby's first steps. The average age for first steps in most countries is around twelve months, although variations from eight or nine months to eighteen months are all considered to be normal. Even though your baby may be able to walk, they may still choose to crawl sometimes, usually because walking is tiring initially, and they can get around quicker using the crawling they have already mastered. They can probably eat independently (albeit messily) with a spoon now and drink from a sippy cup

FUN FACT
When your baby was born, their feet were very underdeveloped, but at twelve months, they are composed of twenty-five constantly growing bones and by the time your child starts school they will have developed into forty-five partially separate bones; these will then fuse to create twenty-six fully developed bones by the time they reach adulthood. It is normal for young children to be flat footed until their feet have finished developing.

independently, and you will notice the fine motor skills involving their hands will rapidly develop, with more and more hand and finger dexterity appearing when they play.

Feeding and eating from nine to twelve months

As your baby becomes more accustomed to eating solid food, they will usually progress to eating three meals a day. You don't need to offer any snacks at this age, but if you think they are still hungry outside of their meals, it is best to offer them more milk. Remember, milk is still the most important source of nutrition for the whole of their first year. At this age, your baby needs to consume around 750 to 850 calories per day, with two-thirds of them still coming from breast or formula milk.

PARENTING Q&A

Q. *Does my baby need 'follow-on milk' now they are older?*

A. *No. Follow-on milk was created as a marketing ploy, to avoid laws prohibiting the advertising of formula milk for babies under six months (also known as 'first-stage formula'). Most formula-milk manufacturers now market milk for babies over six months of age as 'follow-on' milk – not because it is any more appropriate for them, but because it enables them to advertise it. There is no reason to change your baby's formula milk until they are ready to move on to full-fat cow's milk after their first birthday.*

Your baby will now be able to manage finger foods, even if you weaned them using purées. You should still avoid adding salt or sugar to their food and be careful of foods that could pose a choking hazard, such as grapes, which should always be cut lengthways, preferably into quarters, so they cannot get caught in your baby's throat and restrict their airway.

Don't worry if your baby does not like certain foods, as this doesn't mean they will always hate them. The best response to a refused food is to stay calm and just remove it. Try not to bribe or cajole them, as this can impact on their relationship with food as they grow. It can take many repeated exposures to certain foods before a baby is happy to try them, and even

PARENTING Q&A

Q. *Why should babies under twelve months not drink full-fat cow's milk?*

A. *Your baby's nutrition needs are very specific at this age, and regular cow's milk doesn't have all the nutrients they need to grow and develop well. Formula milk is made from cow's milk; however, it has many added ingredients.*

longer for them to like them. It is also quite common for babies to refuse a food they have previously eaten and enjoyed – again, this doesn't mean they will always dislike it. It may just be that they don't fancy it today (just like adults, their preferences for food change daily).

Sleep development from nine to twelve months

While you may be enjoying solid nights of sleep by this point (many nine- to twelve-month-olds do happily sleep through the night), you may also find that your baby is still waking regularly (sadly, just as many don't sleep through). This is also an age when sleep can regress a little, with more night waking and night feeds than you may have experienced just a month or two ago. So what's happening sleep-wise at this stage?

Sleep at nine to ten months

Between nine and ten months, babies sleep for around thirteen hours in every twenty-four-hour period. The average night tops in at ten and a half hours of sleep (remember, you

> **Parent Observation** 'My son's sleep had got into a nice predictable pattern by the time he was about six months old, and we had three joyous months of only one or two night wakes. Then he turned nine months and started waking every two hours. It was exhausting – like being back in the newborn days again! Thankfully, it was fairly short-lived, and we were back to one or two wakes again by his first birthday.'

don't need to deduct time they were awake in the night from this total, just time of bedtime until morning wake time – see page 101). The average nine-month-old will usually have two naps per day, lasting two and a half hours in total. You usually find that one nap (probably the afternoon one) is slightly longer than the other, a common pattern being one hour in the morning and one and a half hours in the afternoon. Although, of course, do remember all babies are unique and it's fine for their sleep patterns to look different. Your baby is now working towards getting most of their sleep at night, as an adult does, with approximately 80 per cent at night and 20 per cent in the day.

As mentioned above, it is not unusual for sleep to regress at this age. You may find your baby wakes up more in the night than they used to, takes longer to settle when they do wake, resists bedtime or needs more milk feeds during the night. All of this is normal and usual at this age and is largely due to separation anxiety (something we will cover in detail in the next section). Research indicates that only 40 per cent of nine-month-old babies sleep in stretches of five or more hours at night, and that the majority are still waking at least once, usually needing parental input to get back to sleep.[6]

Sleep at ten to eleven months

Between ten and eleven months, babies are still sleeping for an average of thirteen hours in every twenty-four-hour period, with a similar split to the previous month of ten and a half hours at night and two and a half in the daytime across two naps. The most common timings for naps to commence are 9.30 a.m. and 2 p.m., with the second one usually lasting longer than the morning one, just as in the previous month.[7] If your baby's sleep regressed a little last month, you may

Anthropology Titbit Although it is the norm for babies to sleep in a cot in their own room in most Westernised countries today, this is historically an unusual sleep set-up. Babies were only moved into their own rooms in the Victorian era. Before this, it was common for children to sleep in the same room as their parents well into toddlerhood. Queen Victoria was famous for her disdain of babies, and she didn't enjoy being around them, as this quote illustrates clearly: 'I have no tender for them till they have become a little human; an ugly baby is a very nasty object and the prettiest is frightful when undressed.'

notice a slight improvement as they approach eleven months; however, increased night waking and feeding are still quite usual at this age. Don't worry, though – it won't last for ever, and their sleep will naturally improve as they get older. Also, any sleep regressions are not because of mistakes you have made – rather, they are a common developmental milestone.

Sleep at eleven to twelve months

As your baby approaches their first birthday, their sleep continues to develop and change. You may find that they start to resist one of their naps a little, and while they are probably not quite ready to drop to one nap per day yet, their resistance is an indication that the transition isn't far off. (We will talk about dropping to one nap more in the next chapter.) By the time babies are eleven months old, their night sleep usually decreases a little, with most now getting around ten hours sleep each night and between two and two and a half hours of daytime naps, still usually split over two naps. Although

FUN FACT

You may notice that your baby sleeps with their eyes open sometimes. This is a fairly common condition, known as nocturnal lagophthalmos, and it affects up to 20 per cent of babies. It is considered medically harmless, although nobody really knows why some babies sleep like this way.

you will hopefully find the effects of the nine- and ten-month sleep regression easing a little by now, over three-quarters of eleven-month-old babies still wake at least once per night and two-thirds of eleven-month-old babies still need at least one night feed.[8]

The average bedtime (that's sleep onset time, not the time you start their bedtime routine) of babies between nine and twelve months is around 8 p.m., with an average wake time of around 7 a.m. Of course, do remember these are average timings, and it is OK for your baby to go to sleep and wake at different times.

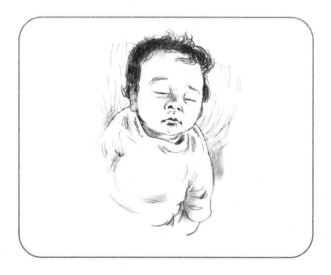

How to improve your baby's sleep
– without sleep training

This is a common time to struggle with your baby's sleep, but there are plenty of little tweaks you can make to their bedtime routines and sleeping environment to positively impact their sleep, without resorting to sleep training. Here are a few ideas:

1. Sleep-friendly lighting
Many parents don't realise that lighting is a key influence on their baby's sleep. Light that is on the blue colour spectrum inhibits melatonin, the hormone of sleep, and tricks the body into thinking it is daytime and thus time to be awake. It isn't just obviously blue light that is an issue, though. Most white light is actually very blue, especially energy-saving light bulbs and halogen spotlights. So too is light that looks green, blue, purple, and pink – which coincidentally tend to be the colours used in most baby night lights. Research has shown that for light to be non-inhibiting it needs to contain very low levels of blue light.[9] Naturally, our ancestors would have illuminated their nights with fire and candles, both sitting on the red colour spectrum. We can replicate this effect by using red light at bedtime and overnight.

2. Bedroom temperature
Our modern homes tend to be well insulated, retaining heat, but this warmth can cause a problem with sleep. The optimal room-temperature range for the best sleep is 15–18°C. Trying to cool the bedroom to somewhere within this optimal range can really help sleep. This doesn't mean

the baby should be cold at night. The aim is 'warm body, cool room'.

3. Humidity

Temperature aside, air conditioning and central heating can cause trouble with sleep in another way, playing havoc with room humidity. Anything that dries the sleeping environment can mean that the baby wakes more for milk because of a dry and sore throat. Where an adult may take a glass of water to place next to their bed, babies tend to wake and cry for milk if they have a dry mouth. This doesn't mean that increasing the humidity will stop the baby needing to feed at night – far from it – but it will remove those extra humidity-related feeds. This tends to be more of an issue for babies who are mouth breathers, sleeping with their mouths open. The best humidity for sleep is around 30–50 per cent. If you do use air conditioning or central heating, you might want to consider placing a humidifier in the bedroom.

4. Night clothes and bedding

Remember 'cool room, warm body' in point two, above? Well, this is where what you dress your baby in at night comes in. Sometimes, adding an extra layer of clothing, such as a long-sleeved vest, or upping the tog rating of a sleeping bag can really help sleep. Generally speaking, in the optimal room-temperature zone (see above), you're looking at a sleeping bag between two and three togs in weight. Some older babies also really hate having their feet covered by anything (unsurprisingly, since we tend to sleep better with our feet exposed). For this reason, you may find it helps to use a sleeping bag with separate leg sections and foot holes.

5. Music

If you sing your baby to sleep or use a mobile or stuffed animal that plays music for fifteen or twenty minutes at bedtime, you could be causing your child to wake more. Why? Remember that babies have very short sleep cycles, lasting for less than an hour, and at the end of a sleep cycle, one of three things may happen: a) they move straight into a new cycle; b) they wake fully and need your help to start a new cycle; or c) they wake ever so slightly, but not fully, and if all is well, they start a new cycle independently. The third scenario is where it is important to consider any constants in the room. If a baby goes to sleep with music, that music needs to be present all night. At the end of a sleep cycle, your slightly rousing baby needs to hear the same sounds as when they went to sleep. If they don't, the sharp change in environment may cause them to wake fully and need your help. Some manufacturers try to get around this by designing noise- and motion-activated music players. These rarely work, however, because they only kick in when the baby is already roused and moving and crying. Consider playing an 'alpha music for children' recording all night. This type of music is recorded to a resting pulse rate of sixty beats per minute and includes elements of white noise, heartbeats and simple repetitive music, all of which aid sleep far more effectively than standard 'sleepy' music. Turn the music on at bedtime and leave it playing until the following morning on a low volume.

6. Scent

The smell in the world that relaxes your baby the most is the smell of you. If you could bottle this and spray it around their bedroom, it would surely comfort them. Many parents pop muslins in their tops to absorb their scent and then leave this with their baby, or one of their T-shirts or pyjama tops. This can work well for some, but other babies need more. To get more, you need to condition a smell. And to do this, you need to take a scent and make it yours. The easiest and most effective way to do so is to select an aromatherapy oil that you like (and is safe to use around babies), such as lavender or chamomile, and pop some of it on as perfume each day for a month or so. Then use it in an aromatherapy diffuser in the room your baby sleeps in for an hour before bedtime.

7. A consistent bedtime routine

Scientists unanimously agree: if there is one thing that has the biggest impact on baby sleep, it is a consistent bedtime routine. While a similar bedtime each night is important for setting the baby's circadian rhythm (body clock), what is more important is doing the same thing in the same order each and every night. For instance, a bath, followed by a massage, followed by a story, followed by a breastfeed or bottle. Try to keep the bedtime routine as calm as possible (it is preparing for sleep, after all) and remember to only use lighting on the red colour spectrum (see point one, above).

8. Bedtime snacks

Once your baby is well established on solids and they are eating three meals a day, you could introduce a small bedtime snack. Aim to give this just before the bedtime routine starts – around an hour before they normally go to sleep. Bedtime snacks can not only fill up tummies that may be hungry, but they can also help from a chemical point of view, and incorporating a snack that contains tryptophan (an amino acid that influences the production of sleep hormones) is a great choice. Baby-friendly sources of tryptophan include cheese, eggs, oats and bread.

Following these tips may not magically encourage your baby to sleep through the night, but they should, hopefully, have a positive impact, without the need to sleep train.

Social and psychological development from nine to twelve months

Months nine to twelve are all about one word for your baby: trust. By this age, they have acquired something known as object permanence, describing their ability to know that something still exists even when they can't see it. For instance, if a beloved toy is hidden in a cupboard, they may become upset because they know that it exists, but they can't see or hold it. Object permanence also tells us that a baby's memory – and their limbic system – is developing, because in order for them to know that something exists that they can't see, they have to remember it and then be upset when they miss it. It is the combination of object permanence, memory and big feelings that form separation anxiety – an entirely normal, but often distressing stage that nine-to-twelve-month-old babies go through.

At this age, your baby knows that you exist, even when they can't see you, and their memory of you triggers feelings of sadness, fear and anxiety when they can't see you because

> Attachment is a deep and enduring emotional bond that
> connects one person to another across time and space.
> *John Bowlby, British psychoanalyst*

they don't understand that you haven't left them for ever. This whole reaction is a wonderful testament to your parenting and the bond you have formed with them. Many people worry that separation anxiety is a sign that their baby is 'clingy' and will always stay that way, but the research shows that babies are meant to cling at this age, and it is their very clinginess that helps them to be confident and independent as they grow.[10]

Attachment theory

In the 1950s and 60s, British psychoanalyst John Bowlby described attachment as a 'lasting psychological connectedness between human beings'.[11] Bowlby's work initially started due to his interest in the impact of separation from their parents on hospitalised children in the period between the First and Second World Wars. From his studies of these children, he formulated his theory of attachment.

Bowlby believed that attachment was important for infants, ensuring their survival because it caused them to constantly seek to be in close proximity to their parent or carer. This sort of attachment is not unique to humans; it can be seen in the behaviour of many mammals and their young, especially primates. Bowlby described the parent or carer as providing a 'secure base' for the baby – a place they could always return to, to feel safe, after exploring the world. (Chapter 6 will expand on the idea of attachment, looking at how it changes in the

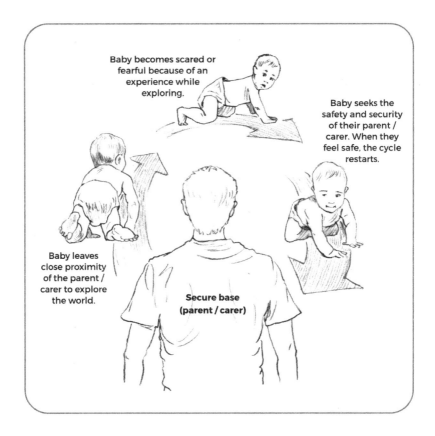

toddler years and how it can affect a child's relationships with others as they move into adulthood.)

Perhaps the strongest indicator of a secure attachment between nine and twelve months is a baby who is comfortable exploring their surroundings when in the presence of their parent, but who then becomes highly upset when they leave.

> Try to prise a limpet away from its rock and it will cling all the harder.
> *Jeremy Holmes, British psychiatrist,*
> *on John Bowlby and attachment theory*

Parent Observation 'Before I understood attachment theory, I thought my son's separation anxiety was a sign that I spent too much time with him, and he needed to be socialised by spending time away from me. I felt so relieved when I realised that it was normal, and I hadn't done anything wrong.'

The best way to help your baby to feel safe and secure, and to encourage confidence and independence as they grow, is to respond to their need for attachment now, by acting as their secure base and allowing them to cling whenever they need to.

Stages of attachment

In the 1960s, psychologists Rudolph Schaffer and Peggy Emerson analysed the attachment behaviours of sixty babies from birth to eighteen months. They identified four main stages of attachment in infancy:

1) **Pre-attachment stage: birth to three months** During this phase, newborns do not display an attachment to a particular adult and rarely show a preference for a specific parent or carer (breastfeeding aside).

2) **Indiscriminate attachment: six weeks to seven months** In this phase, babies begin to show a preference for and attachment to one or two primary carers, but will happily accept care from others, too.

3) **Discriminate attachment: seven to eleven months** At this point, babies begin to demonstrate a strong attachment and preference for one specific carer (usually their mother), demonstrating distress and separation anxiety when away from them.

4) **Multiple attachments: nine months and beyond** In this
   final stage, babies develop attachments with several carers
   and are happy to accept care from other family members
   and childcare workers that they form a bond with.

Note: some of these stages overlap, as infants move through
them at different ages; therefore, there is a range for each.

PARENTING Q&A

Q. *What can I do to help my baby form an attachment to
the nursery staff when I go back to work?*

A. *Most nurseries offer something known as a keyworker
scheme, where one member of staff will work hard
to form a special relationship with your child and be
the main point of contact for you. Setting up several
meetings or trial sessions with the keyworker, yourself
and your baby, before leaving them at nursery, will help
a bond to form. You could also consider sending them
to nursery with a special blanket or muslin that they
associate with you (i.e. one you always hold when you
are cuddling them) and ask their keyworker to hold it
when they need to calm your baby. This will provide a
bridge between you and the keyworker and help your
baby form an attachment with them.*

Language and communication from nine to twelve months

At nine months, your baby will understand some basic words and commands – for instance, 'No', 'Hello', 'Come here' and 'Bye bye', although just because they understand the word 'No' and other related commands, don't expect them to listen![12] Responding to your discipline attempts at this age requires a level of brain development and self-control that they don't yet possess.

It is likely that your baby's first word, or words, will appear during this period, and by the time they reach their first birthday they will probably have two or three in their vocabulary. First words often include 'Hi', 'Bye', 'Cat', 'Dog' and 'No'.

While your baby is busy learning how to talk in their native language, one language-related skill they have lost over

FUN FACT
'Uh oh' are the two most common words strung together by babies once they begin to talk.[13]

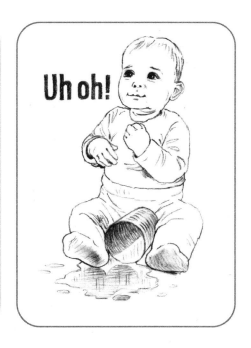

the last three months is the ability to discriminate the sounds of other (non-native) languages.[14] This is a good example of their maturing brain beginning to prune excess synaptic connections that aren't reinforced (see page 184), in order to concentrate on the most important connections – in this case, those involving their own native language (or languages, if you are raising them to be bilingual).

Play ideas for babies from nine to twelve months

Play is not only the primary source of learning at this age, but also a wonderful way for babies who struggle with separation anxiety to form strong attachments with adults other than their primary caregiver. Research observing babies aged nine to fifteen months and their parents during play sessions found that the brains of both the babies and their parents synched when they played together.[15] Scientists have found similar neural activity in the same regions of the brain for both baby and adult during play – an effect known as 'neural synchrony'. Not only did researchers find similarities between baby and adult brain activity, but they also found that the play stimulated areas of the brain responsible for higher functioning, indicating that playing with an adult is an excellent way to encourage more advanced brain development.

Play at this age is ideally focused on developing both gross motor skills (development and co-ordination of large muscles and muscle groups) and fine motor skills (the development of smaller muscle groups and dexterity). Look for activities that encourage movement, such as dancing, and finer skills, such as stacking blocks.

Now your baby has developed object permanence (see page 128), they often enjoy games such as 'peek-a-boo' or searching for hidden objects – for instance, hiding a ball under a cup. Finally, this is a great age to allow them to get messy with their play, allowing them to explore their senses through play.

Recommended toys

As with the other stages thus far, you are still your baby's favourite plaything and any toys you do buy don't need to be expensive or complicated. Babies of this age still prefer simple toys that they can manipulate in many different ways. Here are some top toy recommendations:

- **Stacking cups** – for hiding other objects, pouring in the bath and lining up as well as stacking

- **Wooden blocks** – for banging together and sorting into different colours, as well as stacking

- **Hand puppets** – especially for hiding and playing peek-a-boo with

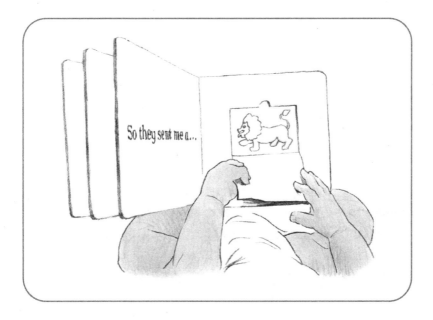

Parent Observation 'No matter how much money we spent on toys, my daughter's favourite thing to play with when she was a baby was an old wooden spoon from our kitchen. The spoon used to come everywhere with us!'

- **Shape sorters** – good for fine motor skills
- **Simple musical instruments**, such as a wooden xylophone for banging or maracas for shaking
- **Board books** with 'lift-the-flap' sections to build on both your baby's literacy skills and their fine motor skills
- **Wooden activity cubes** – especially ones that can be used as a support while your baby learns to stand and cruise; these are great for gross motor skills and also for developing fine motor skills while they enjoy the many different activities on them

At this stage, your baby will probably also like to imitate you and some of your everyday activities – say, with a mobile phone (either a toy or an old, real one). If you do have some everyday objects you are thinking of throwing away, do check if they are safe for your baby to use and play with; they may well end up being some of their favourite toys!

As this chapter comes to an end, we also mark the close of your baby's first year. This is a good time to flip back through the previous chapters to remind yourself of quite how far they have come and to marvel at the new skills they have acquired, before you move on to learning about the year to come in Chapter 6.

6

Twelve to Eighteen Months

Congratulations on your baby's first birthday! Although they are still very much your baby, official definitions now consider them to be a toddler. The American Center for Disease Control (CDC) considers a toddler to be a child aged one to two years, while the parameters according to the British National Health Service (NHS) are twelve to thirty-six months. Toddlers are so named because of their 'toddle'-type walk, but even if your child is not walking yet, they are still considered to be a toddler. My preferred name for children of this age, however, is 'boddler' (from 'baby-toddler'). This term isn't recognised by any official sources but seems to me much more fitting for this age range. At twelve months, they certainly feel more like a baby than a toddler, but by the time they reach eighteen months, there is no doubt that they are fully into the realms of toddlerdom.

How the brain develops from twelve to eighteen months

Your boddler's brain has undergone an immense transition in their first year. Their cerebral cortex (the outermost layer of their brain) has grown by an amazing 88 per cent since they were born. Their prefrontal cortex (the section of the brain involved in higher cognitive processes, such as memory,

Children are not only innocent and curious, but also optimistic and joyful and essentially happy. They are, in short, everything adults wish they could be.
Carolyn Haywood, American writer and illustrator

decision making and attention) is busy creating new synaptic connections, wiring the brain for future, more mature, behaviour over the coming years. Although peak synaptic production occurs in the prefrontal cortex during this stage, it is only in the late teenage years that the brain has a similar number of connections to an adult's.[1] Huge synaptic development is also occurring in areas of the brain responsible for language acquisition, and you will see these connections directly reflected in your boddler's speech and level of understanding over the coming months, as they begin to babble and experiment with sounds more and first words appear.

Your child's brain isn't only busy forming new connections; it is also hard at work on myelination, coating more of its neurons in the fatty substance which helps to speed the electric impulses travelling through it.[2] Myelination at this age is very much concentrated in the parts of the brain involved with language – again, directly reflected in language-acquisition skills. The limbic area of the brain (responsible for

Neuroscience Nugget   If your toddler regularly listens to music, their prefrontal cortex and auditory cortex (the parts of the brain which help to process speech) will be more developed than they are in those who are not regularly exposed to music.[3]

How do you nurture and stimulate your boddler's brain?

You are probably already nurturing and stimulating your little one's brain without even realising – the following really help it to develop to its full potential:

* Providing reassurance when they are upset, or fearful (meeting their needs for connection) and trying to limit stressful situations as much as possible

* Loving touch: hugs, massages and gentle rubs when they hurt themselves

* Encouraging them to get involved with different sensory experiences, stimulating their sense of smell and touch, as well as vision, taste and hearing

* Reading to them as much as possible, trying to include a daily story in their bedtime routine

* Playing music around them, singing with them, encouraging them to enjoy musical instruments

* Talking to them often, gazing into their eyes, smiling, laughing and listening to their responses

* Offering them nourishing foods to eat (but not panicking too much if they are refused)

You are still the biggest positive influence on your child's brain development at this stage; they don't need expensive educational toys or classes – they just need a nurturing, stimulating, encouraging relationship with you and the other adults who care for them.

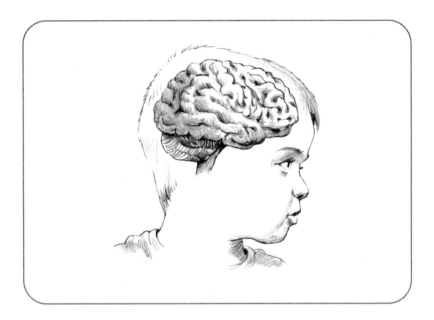

big emotions) is also rapidly myelinating, and this period is, consequently, the most likely time for you to encounter your boddler's first temper tantrum. The maturing limbic system also helps them to gain a sense of self-awareness. They begin to understand who they are and their place in the world, which is often a trigger for tantrums, as they move out of the period of separation anxiety experienced in the previous few months and push for some autonomy and control for the first time.

Using an electro encephalogram (EEG), researchers from the Birkbeck BabyLab in London (a laboratory focused on the developing infant brain) monitored twelve-month-olds,

Neuroscience Nugget Researchers estimate that only 50 per cent of parents read aloud to their children at this age, even though it is one of the best ways to encourage cognitive development.

> *FUN FACT*
> *By the time they are one year old, a baby usually weighs*
> *about three times their birth weight.*

while the toddlers watched videos designed to be specifically engaging to their age group. Results found that brain activity at twelve months could predict the child's intelligence at seven years of age, showing how important these months are for parents and carers to nurture and stimulate their child's growing brain.[4]

Physical development from twelve to eighteen months

Physical development between twelve and eighteen months is very much focused on movements becoming more controlled and refined. Along with this comes speed; if you haven't already done so, by the end of this period you are likely to find yourself rushing after your boddler while they run away from you, delighting in the chase.

Physical milestones: twelve to fifteen months

By the end of this period, your boddler is likely to be able to:

- master walking
- push a toy as they walk (for example, a baby walker)
- throw a ball
- crouch down to pick something up and then stand again

- reach for something and pick it up while standing
- take off their socks and shoes (without laces or complicated buckles)
- show some interest in mark making – using a crayon to create random marks and dots on a piece of paper
- show an interest in climbing.

Physical milestones: sixteen to eighteen months

By the time they are eighteen months, your boddler – or toddler as they will by then definitely be – is likely to:

- learn to walk backwards
- pull a toy behind them as they walk
- become more adept at climbing (on and off furniture, for example) and tackle stairs with your help

PARENTING Q&A

Q. *My sixteen-month-old gets very frustrated when we don't let him take his socks off, but I worry about his feet getting cold.*

A. *Your toddler is working on his fine motor skills, and practising taking off his socks is a great way to develop them. If you're at home, you could incorporate taking off socks into play every day, perhaps encouraging him to see if he can take off your socks or a favourite teddy's. If he does it when you're out and you're worried about him getting cold feet, then pick shoes that he cannot take off independently.*

- help to undress themselves (pulling down elasticated trousers, for example)
- use cutlery as they eat
- stack several blocks
- complete puzzles with two or three large individual pieces
- show greater interest in mark making, producing more controlled back and forward scribbles.

While the first half of this period is concentrated on mastering gross motor skills, the second half focuses heavily on fine motor skills, as your child becomes more and more proficient at using and co-ordinating their hands for more complex tasks.

Anthropology Titbit   Korean families perform a fortune-telling ritual known as Doljabi on their baby's first birthday in which the baby is placed on the floor in front of a range of objects, such as food, paintbrushes, money, wool or thread. According to tradition, the item the child picks indicates their future fortunes. For instance, if they pick money, they will be wealthy as they grow; if they pick the thread, or wool, they will have a long life; if they pick the paintbrush, they will be artistic or creative; and if they pick food, they will not go hungry in life.

Children cannot bounce off the walls if we take the walls away.
Erin Kenny, author and forest school advocate

Why spending time in nature is good for development

Research has shown that children who grow up with regular access to green spaces, such as forests, parks and community gardens, show better development than those who do not.[5]

Spending time in nature encourages your boddler's physical development, giving them space to walk and run, with obstacles to navigate and climb. The freedom of being outside and making as much noise as they want helps communication skills and increases levels of happiness. The sensory input from the different smells, textures, sounds and sights invites them to interact more with the world around them, learning about science, maths and art in a natural way that is entirely open ended. Being outside often also helps a child's developing immune system and can also protect their eyesight, making them less likely to need glasses as they grow.

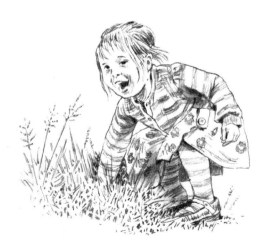

Feeding and eating from twelve to eighteen months

Your boddler is likely well established on solids by now, eating three meals per day. Now that they are one, if they are bottle-fed, they no longer need infant formula and can change on to full-fat cow's milk. It is important to give full-fat milk, as brain development requires fat, plus it provides extra calories for growth. Dentists recommend that from twelve months, if you are bottle-feeding, you should move towards giving milk in a cup (either open, or with a free-flowing, valveless spout), rather than a bottle. This is because cow's milk (including formula milk) is more likely to cause dental caries than breast milk and it tends to pool around the teeth when taken from a bottle, making decay more likely.[6]

By twelve months, fewer than 1 per cent of babies in the UK are breastfed, despite the recommendation from the World Health Organization that breastfeeding continues, alongside solid foods, until two years and beyond.[7] Breastfeeding continues to provide the following benefits after twelve months:

- It forms an important contribution to the child's overall nutritional intake.
- It helps the developing immune system, meaning that breastfed toddlers are less likely to get sick.[8]
- It helps to retain a close maternal bond, especially if mother and child are separated during the day.[9]

The decision to stop breastfeeding is an entirely personal one, and the best time to stop is the when it feels best for your family.

When it comes to eating solid foods, your boddler is becoming a pro at using their pincer grip to pick up smaller items and

Anthropology Titbit In Kenya, where breastfeeding toddlers is the norm, one-third of their calories and daily nutrient intake comes from breast milk.[10]

Parent Observation 'We always used to joke that our daughter wore more food than she ate. She used to be covered – her hair, hands, face. It would go all over her and her highchair, but she's a really good eater now and still as enthusiastic about her food as she was back then.'

may be experimenting with different cutlery. They are likely to get very messy when they eat, but don't worry about teaching them table manners just yet. Getting messy during eating is an important developmental aid. Researchers studying the eating habits of sixteen-month-olds – in particular, how much mess they made, including deliberately squashing food with their hands – found that the messier the children were allowed to get, the better their food-related vocabulary and identification skills were.[11]

Sleep development from twelve to eighteen months

Hopefully, the sleep regression that tends to accompany the arrival of separation anxiety at around nine months is starting to wear off a little by now. While your boddler's sleep should be easier than it was just a few months ago, don't be in a rush to get them sleeping through the night, or worry if they're not. Night waking continues to be normal at this age, with 55 per

Above all else, keep in mind that babies have no agendas; they are not trying to make it hard on you or manipulate you. With such an undeveloped little brain, they are about as close to their genes as any human will ever get and have little control over their behavior.

Dr James McKenna, American professor of anthropology

cent of twelve- to eighteen-month-olds waking at least once per night on a regular basis.[12]

As babies move into toddlerhood, many people think that they should have developed the ability to 'self-soothe' or 'self-settle' when they wake in the night, meaning that whatever the cause of the waking, the child should be able to resolve the problem and start a new sleep cycle without help from their parent or carer. Those potential problems include:

- pain
- being too hot or too cold
- discomfort – such as itching, or a seam or label digging into their skin from their pyjamas
- fear, including nightmares
- separation anxiety
- being hungry or thirsty
- fixing a lighting or noise disturbance.

Having previously discussed what twelve- to eighteen-month-olds are capable of neurologically and physically, it becomes clear that they cannot resolve any of these issues without adult help because their fine motor skills and frontal cortex are not mature enough for the adult-type tasks. Research shows that half of all twelve- to eighteen-month-olds need help from their parents to settle back to sleep when they wake. So does this mean the other half are 'self-settling'?[13] No, it likely means that they are not struggling with a problem that is causing them difficulty with getting to sleep, or back to sleep after they wake.

How do you know when it's time to drop to one nap per day?

The following are signs that your boddler may be ready to drop to a single daily nap:

- Resisting one or both of their naps
- Waking up sooner when they do nap (either for one or both naps)
- Resisting bedtime
- Waking up shortly after going to bed at night
- Waking up earlier in the morning
- Waking more frequently in the night

If you notice at least two of these signs, it is likely that it is time to embrace the nap drop. Instead of keeping one of the original nap times and dropping the other (for example, sticking with one nap at 9.30 a.m. or 2 p.m.), aim to move the remaining one closer to the middle of the day, starting between 11.30 a.m. and 1 p.m. When your boddler is used to the transition, you should find that this nap will last around 90 to 120 minutes, although initially it may be shorter. Don't be misled by normal signs of the transition, such as being overtired and cranky, falling asleep outside of naps and an initial increase in night waking when you drop to one nap. These difficult side effects are only temporary, usually disappearing within two to four weeks.

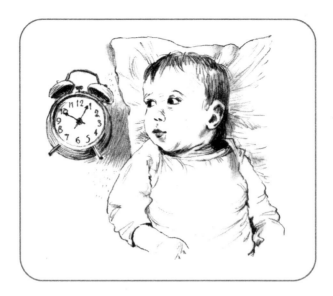

So what should you expect of your twelve- to eighteen-month-old's sleep, aside from needing to help them when they wake in the night? Most boddlers sleep for ten hours at night, with the average bedtime (time of sleep onset, not the time the bedtime routine starts) at around 8.30 p.m. and the average wake time between 6.30 and 7 a.m. Most will drop to one nap per day during this period, usually taken just before or after lunch, with the average length ranging between one and a half and two hours. If they are still taking two naps per day, then each usually lasts for around one hour, generally taken around 9.30 a.m. and 2 p.m.[14]

Social and psychological development from twelve to eighteen months

Social and psychological development between twelve and eighteen months has two main focuses – self-awareness and attachment – and they are closely interlinked. For a boddler to become self-aware (understanding who they are and how they relate to the world) and confident, they have to be securely attached to others. This attachment ultimately gives way to the realisation that they are a unique being (who can be left alone – hence the separation anxiety) and helps them to feel safe and secure as they explore the world and their place in it.

The mirror test

One way of assessing self-awareness in boddlers is using the mirror, or rouge, test. If you mark a dot of colour somewhere on a fifteen-month-old's face (the dot was originally made using rouge – or blusher – hence the alternative name) and then sit them in front of a mirror, most will reach out to the glass and try to touch and wipe off the mark. *After* fifteen months, most will look in the mirror and touch the spot on their face, indicating that they are aware that the mark is on them and, therefore, that they recognise themselves in the mirror.

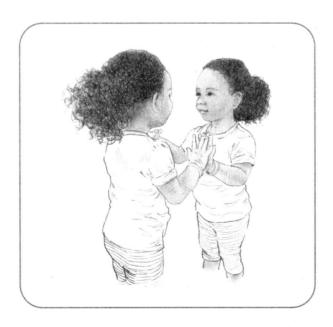

PARENTING Q&A

Q. *When I hurt myself, my fifteen-month-old rushes over and kisses the place in question. Is this a sign that they have an advanced level of empathy for their age?*

A. *Actually, what is more likely happening here is that your child is copying the behaviour they observe from you. For example, if they bump their knee, you will probably give them a hug and rub it better. Rather than having a deep understanding about how you feel, this is more of a conditioned response based on observation. However, it is a great testament to your nurturing parenting.*

Understanding when self-awareness surfaces in childhood helps us to understand the development of other beliefs and emotional behaviour. Self-awareness is necessary before more advanced concepts, such as guilt, regret, shame and empathy, can occur. If children don't have an understanding of themselves, then they cannot possess these feelings, but as self-awareness emerges over the coming months and years, we can expect to see them to some degree.

Ainsworth's strange situation – revisiting attachment theory

In the 1970s, psychologist Mary Ainsworth invented a study to evaluate a baby's attachment to their carer.[15] Ainsworth's work continued the understanding psychologists have of attachment, following Bowlby's idea of the parent providing a 'secure base' from which the child can explore (see page 129). Ainsworth called this experiment the 'strange situation' and it involved children from one to two years entering a room with a parent, then happily playing and interacting normally for a few minutes, before being joined by a stranger. After three minutes with the stranger in the room, the parent exited, leaving the child and stranger alone. Another three minutes passed and then the parent returned to the room and the stranger left. After three minutes more, the parent went out of the room, leaving the child alone. The stranger then returned to the room again. Finally, the experiment was completed with the parent returning and the stranger leaving. In each case, the researchers logged the child's reaction when the parent returned to the room – how much they tried to maintain contact and proximity with the parent, as well as how much comfort the child accepted from them. They also noted how distressed the child was, as well as any happiness shown when the parent returned, and whether the child explored the room or searched for their parent. Based on these observations, researchers classified the child's attachment style as either 'secure', 'resistant' or 'avoidant':

Secure: distressed when the parent leaves the room, searching for them; friendly towards the stranger when the parent is in the room but avoiding them when they are not; happy to explore the room with the parent present, using them as a 'secure base'; happy when the parent returns to the room.

Resistant: extreme distress when the parent leaves the room; avoiding the stranger and fearful of them, even when the parent is also in the room; unhappy to explore the room, even when the parent is present; resistant to reconnecting with the parent when they re-enter the room.

Avoidant: no distress when the parent leaves; happy to interact with the stranger at all points; little notice taken of the parent when they return to the room and just as happy to be comforted by the stranger as the parent.

Ainsworth's work found 70 per cent of children to be securely attached, with the remaining 30 per cent being split equally between resistant and avoidant attachment types. Two decades after this experiment, a fourth attachment style, known as 'disorganised' was added by researchers Main and Solomon.[16] When the parent leaves and enters the room, children with a disorganised style of attachment will act in a confused manner, wandering, looking lost and displaying conflicting behaviours, such as extreme distress at times and nonchalance at others.

What can Ainsworth's work tell us?

The most common and, reassuringly, most positive attachment style is 'secure'. Boddlers (and older children) who are securely attached and exhibit separation anxiety, grow to be emotionally healthier than those with other attachment styles. Secure attachment in the early years is a strong predictor of relationship success in adulthood, impacting all future relationships.[17] The best way to raise your child with a secure attachment is to meet their needs for attachment now.

There are only two lasting bequests we can hope to give our children. One of these is roots. The other is wings.
Hodding Carter, American journalist

Language and communication from twelve to eighteen months

Language is coming on in leaps and bounds now, although you may not necessarily hear the fruits of this development just yet. This is because 'receptive language' (when children listen to words and understand their meaning) is far more developed at this age than 'expressive language' (what they say, or the verbalisation of their understanding). Children's expressive-language skills are still dramatically increasing, and it will take another few months to really hear the results.

Your boddler's speech will develop in four main stages:

1. Babbling

2. Single-word

3. Two-word

4. Multi-word.

They have already mastered stage one and are working hard on stage two at this point.

Two other stages of language development that you may notice at this point are holophrasic speech and overextension.

Holophrasic speech is a term used to describe a boddler's use of certain words (or their own version of them) in place of a whole sentence. For instance, they may say 'apple', or simply 'app', instead of 'I want an apple'. They may even say 'app'

FUN FACT

By the time your baby is eighteen months old, they will be able to understand about ten times more than they can say.

> **Parent Observation** 'When he just started speaking, our son used to call all men "Dada". It was quite embarrassing when we were out in public and he was greeting strange men as "Dada", but thankfully, it only lasted for a few months!'

when they want something to eat (not just an apple), which leads us to the next point.

Overextension refers to when children use a word to describe several different objects which are similar. So in the case of the holophrasic speech example above, if they are hungry and would like a banana, they may still say 'app' because 'app' is their term for all fruit, or even all snacks. Another common overextension example is the use of 'cat' or 'dog' to describe all animals on four legs. This occurs usually because your boddler learns the word for your pet, or an animal they see regularly, and presumes that all other animals are the same. As they grow, their understanding and expressive language will mature, and they will eventually use the correct terminology. Until that happens, just gently use the correct word ('that's a banana') to help them to learn.

Play ideas for twelve to eighteen months

Play during these months will focus on developing fine motor skills. Children are likely to enjoy opening and closing, carrying and stacking things, turning pages of books and exploring their environment with their new-found mobility skills. At this age, you may find that your boddler is happy to potter around by themselves for a few minutes, with some emerging independent play skills. They also like to mirror your actions, copying you putting on your shoes, doing some housework or brushing your hair, for instance.

By observing your little one's natural interests, you will be able to find playthings that entertain them for the longest periods of time. The most popular ones at this age are those that are open-ended (i.e. don't have a limited number of functions) and mirror the real world.

Recommended toys

- **Baby-wipe packets** Recycle an old baby-wipe packet and fill it with cotton handkerchiefs or cut-up muslin squares. Your boddler will enjoy emptying the packet and trying to put the 'wipes' back into the packet.
- **Busy boards** These are homemade toys, created from a sheet of ply- or similar wood, with a selection of doorknobs, handles, locks, door-latch chains, Velcro fastenings, belt clips, wheels on castors, fidget spinners and the like firmly attached. This can either be played with on the floor (and stored under your sofa) or fixed to the wall, if you have space, so your boddler can stand to play with it. Busy boards can be made very easily from items you have lying around the house and are brilliant for encouraging fine motor skills.
- **Puzzles** Wooden puzzles with a few pieces are likely to be of interest now, especially the shape-sorter type.
- **Animal flashcards and matching animal toys** Matching the toy with the animal picture is a popular activity.
- **Finger and hand painting** This is a lovely age to introduce painting – skipping the brushes and going straight for making patterns with their hands provides a brilliant sensory experience for children.

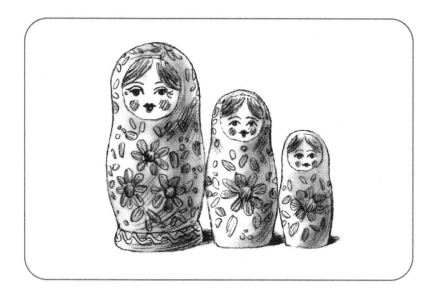

- **Russian-doll-type toys** Your boddler will enjoy unpacking and stacking the pieces back together again.
- **Stacking rings** These have limitless play potential – they can be stacked on the holder, they can be rolled along the floor, they can be sorted by colour, and they are great rolled in paint to create lines on paper.

As these months draw to a close, your boddler is completing the transition from baby to toddler. By the time they are eighteen months old, there is no doubting that they have firmly entered into the world of toddlerhood. It's a bittersweet time: gone is your cuddly little baby, now replaced by an inquisitive and funny ball of energy who is into anything and everything. The toddler years bring fresh challenges, many of which we will cover in the next two chapters, but they bring endless joy and laughter, too.

7

Eighteen to Twenty-four Months

Welcome to toddlerhood! As your child nears the end of their second year they are changing rapidly, physically their motor skills – both gross and fine – are maturing to the point that they are capable of activities similar to an adult. Their language – both receptive and expressive (see page 154) – is exploding and their personality is shining through. Psychologically, this is a time of big change, as your toddler seeks more independence – a testament to the secure base you have provided for them for the last year and a half. This almost never-ending quest for independence, when combined with the brain development typical of this stage, is also the main source of 'fuel' for the tantrums that tend to accompany this period. Starting with an understanding of your toddler's brain is the best way to help you cope with the behaviour that is typical for this stage.

How the brain develops from eighteen to twenty-four months

Your toddler's brain is still growing and developing rapidly, creating new connections every second. The experiences they have with you, and the wider world, will play a huge part in how their brain wires. But it isn't huge, extraordinary events

> **Neuroscience Nugget** When your child reaches twenty-four months, their brain will likely weigh between 1 and 1.1 kg – that's about 10 per cent of their total body weight. And by the time your toddler reaches their second birthday, their brain will be 75 per cent of its full-grown, adult size.[1]

that matter the most; rather, it is the everyday interactions taking place between you and them that will shape who they become.

The neurological emphasis of this age continues to be on language, sensory-related developments and emotions. Towards the end of this period, your toddler's brain will shift focus a little to their prefrontal cortex (responsible for higher cognitive skills, such as impulse control and emotion regulation). This area of the brain will take at least another twenty years to reach maturity, however – not only because of the synaptogenesis and myelination that still has to occur, but also because of a huge amount of neural pruning that will happen throughout the rest of childhood.

At this age, your toddler is full of big feelings, but has little control over them. Their limbic system, or their ability to feel all the feelings, is like a sports car: engine roaring and burning rubber as it travels at full speed. These feeling are so intense that their metaphorical brakes stand no chance when it comes to controlling them. The frequent tantrums, whining, physical violence (hitting, kicking, throwing and so on) that so often accompany toddlerhood are anything but naughty behaviour. In fact, they are caused by neurological development, or rather a lack of it in the area where it is most needed. Your toddler can no more control their outbursts than they can drive a racing car.

A child's mind is not a container to be filled, but rather
a fire to be kindled.
Dorothea Brande, American writer and journalist

Even though toddlers are lacking emotion-regulation skills at this age, what they experience during this period will form their future emotion-regulation control. The way they are treated by parents and carers will impact on the growth, connection and, later, pruning of their prefrontal cortex. So while we can't make a toddler control their behaviour at this age, we can control our own, which, in turn, will help them to learn to control theirs as they grow.

Physical development from eighteen to twenty-four months

Your toddler's gross and fine motor skills develop rapidly between eighteen and twenty-four months. By the end of this period, your toddler is likely to be able to do the following:

- Walk up and down stairs, holding your hand
- Run
- Stack several blocks (usually between four and six)
- Propel themselves forwards on a ride-on toy
- Jump (initially, they are likely to land on one foot, then the other, like a gallop, progressing to landing on both feet by their second birthday)
- Throw a ball (usually underarm at first, then overarm)
- Try to catch a ball, using their whole arms (not just hands)

Parent Observation 'My daughter became obsessed with drawing as soon as she hit eighteen months, and it was always a great way to entertain her. The only problem was she would scribble on everything the minute we turned our backs, and she became a pro at hunting out crayons and pens if we ever left them out.'

- Kick a football
- Squat to pick something up from the floor, or during play
- Make marks on paper (random scribblings at first, but becoming more controlled as they reach their second birthday)
- Use cutlery in a more controlled way (using a spoon to scoop up breakfast cereal, for example)
- Wash and dry their own hands
- Put on and take shoes off with basic Velcro straps

One huge milestone that your toddler will be approaching during this period is potty-training readiness. While most children will be ready to potty train from a physical development point of view around their second birthday, emotionally it may take a little longer for them to be ready to ditch nappies.

Anthropology Titbit In the 1940s, most toddlers were potty trained before eighteen months. The invention of disposable nappies in 1948 and their mass availability in the 1960s have seen a dramatic increase in the average age for potty training to an average age of around three years today.

Signs of potty-training readiness

If you recognise one or two signs from the following list, then it is likely your toddler's mind and body are approaching potty-training readiness:

* They communicate simple body sensations to you (for example, they may say 'I'm hot' or 'I'm hungry').
* They tell you that they need to go to the toilet before they go.
* They can follow a chain of two or three simple instructions – for instance, 'Go get your shoes. Now put your shoes on.'
* They sometimes ask to have their nappy changed or bring you a new nappy when they have soiled their current one.
* They are mostly dry when they wake from a nap.
* Their nappy remains dry for two hours or more at a time.

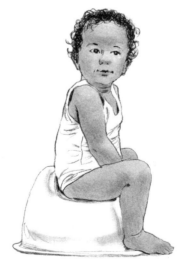

FUN FACT
Your toddler will have got through around five thousand
nappies by the time they are potty trained.

Physiologically, your toddler's bladder needs to grow to hold more urine and their sphincters (muscles responsible for squeezing out and holding in urine and faeces) must develop to the point where they have conscious control over them. These things have usually happened by the time a toddler is somewhere between twenty and thirty months old. Psychologically, your toddler will need to be able to understand their body's signs and communicate their toileting needs, whether verbally or through other cues; they also need to be motivated to lose their nappies and use the toilet. This emotional maturity can take a little longer to develop than the physical.

Feeding and eating from eighteen to twenty-four months

By the time your child reaches eighteen months, they are likely to be an accomplished eater. It is not uncommon for boddlers to eat a huge range of food, including many different vegetables. This easy-eating stage tends to lull parents and carers into a false sense of security, though – because when toddlerhood hits in full force, so do picky and fussy eating.

Toddlers are naturally neophobic, meaning they are scared of and reluctant to eat foods that are unfamiliar. Neophobia is nature's way of keeping toddlers safe, and while this innate protection is not needed so much today, in hunter-gatherer societies toddlers would have been exposed to many

Managing picky and fussy eating

It can be hard not to take your toddler's picky and fussy eating personally. Many parents question what they did wrong to turn their 'good-eater' baby, who ate anything that was put in front of them, into such a fussy toddler. And the answer is: nothing. This is common and normal. It won't last for ever, although it does tend to last longer than parents and carers expect. So what's the best way to manage picky eating?

• **Take off the pressure.** Don't pressure your toddler to eat everything and don't place pressure on yourself either to produce gourmet food that they will love.

• **Give your toddler more control over their eating.** Let them select food from a serving bowl, rather than dishing up everything onto their plate. Or consider using a grazing tray – a plate or tray containing pre-prepared foods that they can help themselves to throughout the day. This way, as the adult, you control what food is presented to your toddler, but they control whether they eat it, and how much.

• **Hold back on the praise and restrict rewards.** It can be tempting to try to bribe your toddler to eat, particularly vegetables and other foods considered to be healthy, but this is likely to place too much emotion on eating, and they can learn to link feeling good (through rewards and praise) with eating more. As they grow, this behaviour can turn into comfort eating and a difficult relationship with food, whereby it is strongly linked with emotions.

- **Be a role model.** Try to eat with your toddler as much as possible, so that they can see you eating and mirror your actions. Don't forget, if you have any strange eating quirks (say, pulling the crusts off of sandwiches), they are likely to copy you.
- **Involve them in food preparation.** Get cooking with your toddler. This is a great age to get your little one fully involved in the kitchen.
- **Let them get messy.** Don't rush to wipe away mess or tell them to keep their hands out of their food. Eating is a very sensory process and research has shown that toddlers who are allowed to get messy when they eat are better eaters; plus, it also improves their learning about the scientific properties of foodstuffs, such as texture and temperature.[2]

dangerous foodstuffs and neophobia prevented them from accidentally ingesting something poisonous. Modern society has evolved hugely with food safety, but neophobia in young children hasn't caught up yet, so when a toddler refuses a new food, rather than being deliberately awkward, they are demonstrating an important evolutionary throwback. Most children will have developed a degree of food neophobia before their second birthday, and many also begin to refuse foods that

FUN FACT
Nearly half of all children are picky eaters at some point in their early years.[3]

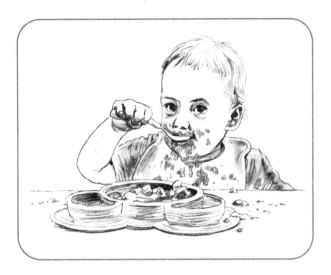

they previously ate happily. The refusal of previously eaten foods may be related to their immature memory development in that they do not remember previously liking the food and therefore neophobia wins out when they refuse it.

As well as through neophobia, nature protects young children from being accidentally poisoned by making toxic foods unpalatable. As discussed in previous chapters, babies favour sweet and savoury tastes, and they tend to dislike sour and bitter flavours. Unsurprisingly, most poisonous substances have a bitter taste. So toddlers' innate taste preferences help to keep them safe by preventing them from accidentally ingesting foods that could endanger their lives, in a similar way to neophobia. Toddlers will often struggle with green

Anthropology Titbit In India, a popular meal for babies and toddlers is khichdi. A one-pot dish made from lentils (dal) and rice, with turmeric and ghee (clarified butter), it is cooked until it has a porridge-type consistency.

PARENTING Q&A

Q. *Does my toddler need a vitamin supplement?*

A. *The NHS recommends that all toddlers are given a vitamin supplement containing vitamins A, C and D every day. Talk to a pharmacist in a local chemist to see which one is best for your toddler.*

vegetables in particular. This is because they contain gluco-sinolates – bitter-tasting compounds that can sometimes be toxic. Safe glucosinolates naturally occur in broccoli, cabbage, kale, Brussels sprouts and many other green vegetables, but toddlers don't understand that they are safe, because of the bitter warning that their taste buds receive, so they tend to avoid eating them.

All toddlers are naturally averse to bitter tastes, but some find them much harder to tolerate than others. In fact, some adults also struggle significantly with bitter-tasting food. Perhaps you do? This is because genetically, some people taste bitter compounds much more strongly than others. Science refers to these individuals as 'strong tasters' and they make up around a quarter of the population (both adult and child). A strong-taster toddler is even more likely to reject vegetables.

Sleep development from eighteen to twenty-four months

Your toddler may well be sleeping more predictably by this time. The average eighteen-month-old gets about thirteen and a half hours' sleep in a twenty-four-hour period. Around

Signs that your toddler may be ready to drop their daytime nap

While most toddlers continue to nap until some point between their second and third year, it isn't uncommon for them to be ready to drop their nap from about twenty months. The following are signs that this may be the case:

- They start to resist their nap.
- They start to resist bedtime.
- They start to wake more in the night.
- They start to wake earlier in the morning.
- Their naps become much shorter, or they wake regularly halfway through and need settling back to sleep.

When your toddler drops their nap completely, it's likely that their night sleep will get worse initially, while their body gets used to taking all sleep at night. Similarly, their behaviour in the daytime may worsen and they may seem very grumpy and overtired. These side effects usually last between two to four weeks, until they adjust to the change in sleep schedule.

FUN FACT

Research into children's language development found that children who listened to the same story at bedtime each night were quicker to learn words in the book than those who had a different one read to them each night.[4]

one and a half to two and a half hours of this occurs during the day, usually in one nap. Do remember, however, that these figures are only an average, and research has shown that some eighteen-month-olds get as few as eleven hours sleep in a twenty-four-hour period (meaning as little as nine hours at night if they have a two-hour nap), while others need as many as sixteen hours (meaning a whopping fourteen hours at night if they still take a two-hour nap).[5] In fact, the most predictable thing about toddler sleep is that it looks different for every child.

By the age of two, most toddlers have dropped a little sleep, to around thirteen hours' total sleep in a twenty-four-hour period, with research showing the range of total sleep as being between ten and fifteen hours.[6] While most toddlers are still napping for one hour in the daytime at this stage, 82 per cent of eighteen- to twenty-four-month-olds have started to skip naps on some days.[7]

PARENTING Q&A

Q. *Is there such a thing as an eighteen-month sleep regression?*

A. *Although there is technically no such thing as an eighteen-month sleep regression, many toddlers do struggle with their sleep during this time period. This is caused by many different things, including new eating patterns, nap drops, potty training, changes in daily routines (for instance, starting nursery) and psychological development (especially related to emotion regulation, emerging independence and attachment).*

Anthropology Titbit The Efé people, from the Ituri rainforest in the Democratic Republic of Congo, do not have specific bedtimes for their children. The whole family stays up together, as long as there is something interesting them, such as a conversation, a dance or a song. Children are free to fall asleep during this entertainment, but they are not told to go to bed by their parents.

Bedtimes tend to get later in toddlerhood, with the average sleep onset time for this age being around 9 p.m.[8] (Remember, this is not when their bedtime routine begins, but the time they are actually asleep.) Night waking is still common in toddlerhood, with research indicating that almost a third of children still wake regularly at night at this age.[9] But the good news is that it shouldn't be long now until this improves.

Social and psychological development from eighteen to twenty-four months

During this period, you may well find yourself wondering what happened to your happy, good-natured baby? Toddlerhood is all about big feelings (the realm of the limbic system) which, combined with a lack of prefrontal cortex brain development, and the resulting lack of emotion-regulation capabilities, brings about the perfect storm most of us refer to as a tantrum.

So what is a tantrum? First off, you should understand that despite frequently being referred to as 'toddler tantrums', they can happen at any age, right into adulthood. The term is simply used to describe the state of an individual (baby,

Parent Observation 'My little boy was so calm and placid, so it was a real shock when he started to tantrum just before his second birthday. I found it hard to deal with his behaviour at first, as I thought it was because I was bad at disciplining him. Understanding what he was going through really helped me to empathise with him, rather than get angry at him. I can't say I'm perfect at that now, but I'm getting better!'

toddler, older child or adult) who is out of control, full of big emotions and stress hormones and unable to calm themselves down and act in a socially acceptable way. As adults, we have largely become adept at managing our own emotions, or at least when we're out in public. Our brains are fully developed, and we have the cognitive skills necessary to calm ourselves down or, rather, 'self soothe'. Toddlers don't possess these skills – not yet anyway. They are not being naughty or manipulative. They are simply being toddlers. Tantrums are a normal and exceedingly common feature of child development. Research has found that 87 per cent of eighteen- to twenty-four-month-olds regularly have tantrums, with most having at least one every day, lasting, on average, between thirty and sixty seconds (although it is not unusual for them to occur far more frequently and last for much longer).[10]

Understanding your toddler's tantrum triggers

A tantrum is like the tip of an iceberg; what you see is the physical manifestation of difficult feelings that your toddler is experiencing. The illustration overleaf shows just some of the potential underlying triggers.

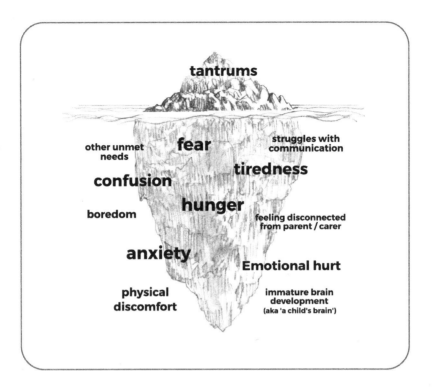

At the root of every tantrum and power struggle are
unmet needs.
Marshall B. Rosenberg, American psychologist

Bion's theory of containment

In the 1960s, an English psychoanalyst named Wilfred Bion
introduced his idea of containment: a concept describing
the way in which parents or primary caregivers are able to
hold space for a child's big, difficult feelings – those which
their brains are not mature enough to manage alone. So
while the child reflects dysregulated behaviour, such as anger,
frustration and anxiety during a tantrum, the parent reflects

What's the best way to tackle a tantrum?

Contrary to popular belief, ignoring, shaming or punishing tantrums can make a toddler's behaviour much worse. Why? Because these approaches ignore the difficult underlying feelings and do nothing to help the toddler to regulate their behaviour or resolve the cause of the tantrum. We have previously learned that babies' and toddlers' brains are affected by the level of parental nurturance they receive. More nurturance, including during a tantrum, means the part of the brain responsible for emotion regulation becomes bigger and better connected as the child grows. If toddlers are constantly sat on naughty steps, sent to time out, punished or ignored when they are perceived to be 'naughty', they do not benefit from the external regulation that the adult provides and, in the long term, will lack the neurological maturity that develops as a result of the nurturance and guidance. The best way to tackle tantrums is as follows:

1. Try to identify and reduce triggers, to prevent tantrums where you can.
2. Keep the toddler (and others) safe during the tantrum.
3. Stay calm and hold your boundary; supporting and nurturing isn't about giving in.
4. Help your toddler to calm down once the tantrum is over. The best way to do this is to mirror calmness yourself.

You cannot stop tantrums. And they are not a sign of poor parenting. Remember, they are a normal stage of child development, caused by immature brain development. In time your toddler will grow out of them, until then understanding and a lot of patience is the best way forward.

calmness, control and regulation, helping the child to become calmer. The theory of containment is why staying calm and supportive during a tantrum is so important.

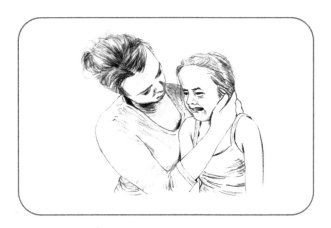

PARENTING Q&A

Q. *My toddler's favourite words at the moment are 'me do it'. If I don't let her do whatever it is, then she has a huge tantrum. What can we do?*

A. *Toddlers really struggle with a desire for independence and an innate drive for autonomy at this age. It's all part of growing up and the start of them learning to be confident without you. As important as it is, it is also incredibly frustrating! The answer is to give your toddler as much control as possible over areas of her life where it's age appropriate. For instance, allowing her to choose her own clothes in the morning, letting her direct her own play and giving her choices at mealtimes. The more control she is given by you, the less she will feel frustrated and tantrum.*

Language and communication from eighteen to twenty-four months

The period between eighteen and twenty-four months sees a real language explosion. Your toddler likely says around ten to twenty words at eighteen months, but by the time they reach twenty-four months, the average toddler has a vocabulary of between fifty and one hundred words, and some even approach two hundred words.

As well as a growing vocabulary, toddlerhood sees your child beginning to string two words together into simple

PARENTING Q&A

Q. *My son started to stutter just before his second birthday. He doesn't do it all the time but seems to get stuck on some words sometimes. Is this normal?*

A. *Stuttering commonly appears between eighteen and twenty-four months, affecting between 5 and 10 per cent of toddlers. It often coincides with the language explosion that takes place at this stage. It is thought that stuttering largely occurs when a toddler's busy brain cannot clearly express their thoughts. In a sense, it's almost as if their brains are working faster than their mouths. Most toddlers will outgrow their stuttering naturally; until they do, it's best to stay calm and patient while they speak and avoid trying to complete words or sentences for them. If you are concerned that the stuttering is not passing, do speak with your family doctor.*

FUN FACT
Toddlers who are regularly spoken to by their parents learn about three hundred more words by the age of two years, than those whose parents speak to them less.

sentences, such as 'Hello, Daddy' and 'Want snack'. They are more likely to initiate conversation at this age, rather than simply replying when you speak to them and, increasingly, they will accompany their words with gestures, too.

Your toddler has always understood more than they can say, but this understanding of language is also expanding now. They can follow simple verbal cues, such as 'Get your shoes' and will also be able to point to relevant parts of their body when you say things such as 'Where's your arm?'

The best ways to boost your toddler's language skills are similar to previous stages: speaking with them regularly, reading stories daily, especially at bedtime, and using the correct names for people and objects.

Play ideas for eighteen to twenty-four months

As your toddler masters gross motor skills and their fine motor skills continue to develop, there are many new play ideas and toys to choose from. This is also a lovely age to encourage your child's imagination and to engage in the world of make believe, with puppets and something known as 'small-world play'.

Small-world play involves using toys to act out real-life scenarios and stories from books or similar. For instance, your toddler may love to play with toy animals and act out a scene

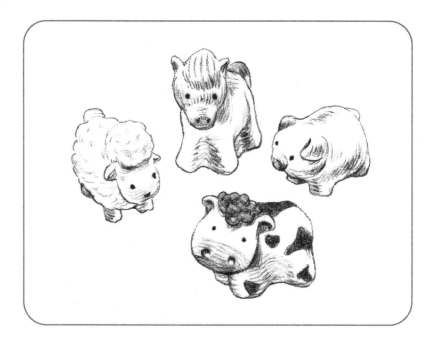

from a zoo or a farm they have visited. Or they may like to create a city scene to drive cars around. Small-world play is wonderful not only for stimulating your toddler's imagination, but also for building their fine motor skills. From a parent or carer's perspective, it has great value – both financially, because you can use many everyday objects, and from a time perspective, as it often holds a toddler's attention for longer than conventional toys.

Here are some suggested small-world set-ups:

- Use a large cardboard box to create a town – you can draw roads and buildings on it, for your toddler to drive cars around.

- A builder's tray or 'tuff tray' can be filled with sand, shells, pebbles and an old ice-cream tub containing water to create a beach scene, complete with toy fish in a rock pool.

- Fill an old ice-cream tub with water, add some polar animals (like polar bears and penguins) and freeze. When it is solid, cut away the tub and put it in a builder's tray or tuff tray for your toddler to play with as the ice melts.

- Pick some grass and flowers, sticks, pine cones and similar from your garden or a nearby park and use toy insects or animals to create a farm or forest scene for your toddler to play with.

The beauty of small-world-play ideas is that there is no limit to what you can create with very little money and few toys. And it is easy to change the 'world', or theme, to keep the play fresh for your toddler.

Recommended toys

- **Ride-on toys** At this age toddlers will often be interested in ride-on toys, such as mini scooters and cars. These also help them with movement co-ordination.

- **Threading** A lovely, inexpensive activity, often using items you have lying around the house – such as pasta or large beads and string – to practise fine motor skills.

- **Make believe** Many toddlers enjoy make-believe items, such as puppets and dolls, often using them to act out stories or mimic your actions – for instance, caring for a doll if there is a new baby in the family.

- **Building blocks** Many toddlers of this age are fascinated with building blocks, from wooden shapes to plastic bricks, such as Duplo.

- **Peg boards** These are great for little fingers to practise fine motor skills by putting pegs in the holes.

- **Jigsaw puzzles** Go for either wooden puzzle pieces or chunky board puzzles that will survive little hands.
- **Arts and crafts** This is a lovely age to introduce more craft equipment, such as Play-Doh, crayons and paint.

As your toddler's first 1,001 days (from conception through to their second birthday, deemed by many as the most important days in their life) come to an end, this is a good time to take stock of the last two years and to reflect on quite how much they have achieved, with your help. Parents and carers can sometimes be very self-critical, berating themselves for not being good enough or stimulating their child enough. Hopefully, this chapter (and all those before) has shown you what a wonderful job you are doing and what a great job you will continue to do as your child grows. Let's move on now to looking at the year ahead from your toddler's second to third birthday – because although you have got used to counting your toddler's age in months, years will be the focus for development from this point on.

8

Two to Three Years

Welcome to 'the terrific twos'! Usually this time frame is more commonly known as 'the terrible twos', but there is nothing terrible about your child at this age. Your two-year-old is a wonder of nature; their development – neurologically, physiologically and psychologically – is a marvel. Yes, they will tantrum, but to define them by their tantrums – or immature brain development – does them a great disservice. This chapter will shed light on the wonders of this age and, hopefully, get you excited at everything you have to look forward to with your little one.

How the brain develops from two to three years

Your toddler's brain is still busy creating new synaptic connections. During this year, the density of synapses in their prefrontal cortex (responsible for higher cognitive skills, such as reasoning and impulse control) is around 200 per cent of the final adult volume. Myelination continues, but despite this rapid development, the prefrontal cortex is still incredibly immature, lacking the finely honed, fast connections you find in an adult's brain, occurring only through repeated experiences and careful pruning. A toddler's prefrontal cortex connections are rather like the drawer that everybody has at home, storing a tangled ball of unused cables and chargers, just in case you'll need them one day. They are full of wires and potential connections, but rather jumbled and difficult to find what you're looking for. To make use of the cables, you need to carefully sort through them, checking the connections and discarding those that no longer serve you or are too slow. This slow, careful process leaves a streamlined collection of the fastest wires, akin to a mature adult prefrontal cortex.

While you can expect your toddler to show some increase in their cognitive skills and more flexibility in their thinking – in particular, a new-found ability to comprehend cause and effect and to understand and interpret events, both past and present – their brain is still nothing like that of an adult.[1] Your toddler still exists very much in the world of the limbic brain (the area of big emotions) spending very little time in the world of the prefrontal cortex.

Synaptic pruning

While a toddler's brain is busy creating new synaptic connections, this period also sees the beginning of synaptic pruning. This is a little like pruning rose bushes, snipping away the dying blooms, so that the plant can grow stronger and create bigger, brighter ones in the future. In the case of pruning – or removing – synaptic connections, your toddler's brain is ensuring that it can be as effective as possible. Older, weaker, synaptic connections are pruned to make way for new ones and to strengthen those already in existence through repeated use.

Neuroscience Nugget At birth, the number of synapses per neuron is 2,500, but by age two or three, it's about 15,000.[2]

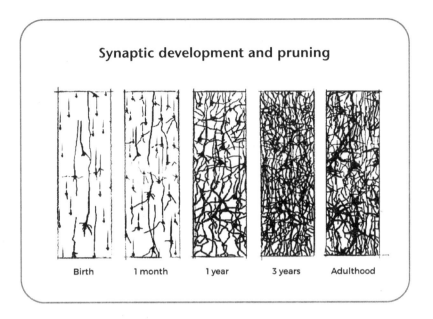

Synaptic development and pruning

Birth   1 month   1 year   3 years   Adulthood

By the time your child is ten years old, synaptic pruning will have removed about 50 per cent of the extraneous synapses in their brain, leaving the connections as streamlined and as fast as possible. The diagram above shows just how quickly synapses develop in the first three years of life, and how they decrease, through pruning, as children grow.

Physical development from two to three years

You will notice that your toddler's weight gain slows now, with them putting on around 0.2kg per month, as opposed to almost half a kilogram per month in the early toddler period.

You will likely notice that your toddler is a lot steadier on their feet in this age range, probably enjoying running and jumping and increasingly confident in their new-found climbing skills. They will start to favour an overarm technique when they throw a ball, and can now kick a ball and aim in a rough

> ### FUN FACT
> *A child's height on their second birthday is usually roughly half of their final adult height.*

direction. Your toddler is also experimenting with balance and may be able to stand on one leg and lift the other off of the floor for a few seconds.

Physical milestones

Physical milestones at this age focus on fine motor skills and by the end of this period, your toddler is likely to be able to:

- hold a crayon with something known as a 'digital pronate grasp' (whereby they hold the crayon with their fingers and palm pointing downwards)
- draw with controlled scribbles, featuring backward and forward lines, rough circles and dots
- begin learning how to snip (rather than accurately cut) paper with a pair of children's scissors
- string large wooden beads onto thick thread
- build a tower of six to eight blocks
- pick up small objects from the floor
- turn individual pages of a book
- climb up onto and then jump off a low object, such as a chair
- take off most items of clothing (without complicated buttons and zippers) independently
- put on their socks and shoes (without laces)

- start to tackle big buttons on their clothing independently
- use cutlery more efficiently to eat their food (though still get messy!).

This period is all about your toddler learning to become independent. The more they can do for themselves, the more they

---

How to give your toddler more autonomy

- Allow them to choose their own clothes (you can sort their wardrobe to be season appropriate) where possible.
- Allow them to dress themselves when you're not in a rush.
- Give them more control over their eating, by using a serving dish and letting them serve food onto their own plate.
- Set up a snack station and a small water dispenser, so they can get help themselves whenever they're hungry or thirsty.
- Encourage them to choose a book to read every day with you.
- Allow them to direct you in playtime for a few minutes each day.
- Encourage them to help you with household tasks – for instance, let them use a dustpan and brush to sweep the floor.
- Give them opportunities to get more involved in their own body care – such as brushing their teeth and washing their hands independently, using a step to stand on to reach the sink.

PARENTING Q&A

Q. *How do you know whether your child is right- or left-handed? My daughter sometimes favours her right hand, but she will still use both hands interchangeably most of the time.*

A. *Most children will show a preference for using their right or left hand by the time they are two years old, with definite right- and left-handedness showing by three years of age. Around 90 per cent of three-year-olds are right-handed, 9 per cent are left-handed and 1 per cent are ambidextrous (use both hands equally).*

will grow in confidence and self-esteem. They will thrive on being given more autonomy; many tantrums at this age are due to toddlers struggling with a lack of control over their lives, so it follows that the more control you give them, the less likely it is that they will tantrum.

Feeding and eating from two to three years

Picky and fussy eating are still very common during this period. It is likely that your toddler will be fickle in their eating, happily eating a specific food with gusto one week, then turning their nose up at it as if it were poisonous the next. This is not an indication that you have done something wrong as a parent, nor is it a sign that they will always be picky. Toddler eating is complicated. They are still highly neophobic (refusing unknown foods) and eating is also a way for them to control the world around them, so at times when they feel out of control you will often find that they become even more picky. Eating is also an incredibly sensory experience for your toddler, and although many love to get mucky, with food and other substances, some will really struggle with different textures, particularly slimy foods and those in sauces. Finally, the world is highly exciting for your toddler, and eating often means being dragged away from something far more interesting and important to them – play!

The best way to cope with tricky eating during toddlerhood is to stay calm, keep presenting foods that have been previously refused and offer a safe (quick-to-prepare) alternative you know they will eat as a fallback. Eating can quickly become a battle between toddler and parent or carer, but it is a battle that neither will win so it's best avoided in the first place.

Table manners

Your toddler is likely to have grown out of their highchair by this age and has probably joined you at the table in a booster seat. It can be tempting to expect them to sit at the table and join in at mealtimes like adults, but their immature brain development prevents this from happening. Toddlers have short attention spans. Once they have finished, they quickly get bored sitting at the table and don't care if others are still eating. They will want to get down, and if they are not allowed to do so (or at least to play with toys while sitting there), then a tantrum is likely to ensue. This behaviour isn't 'naughty' or 'antisocial', and it certainly isn't a sign that they will grow up to be lacking in table manners. Remember, the limbic system in their brain allows them to feel big emotions, but their prefrontal cortex doesn't yet enable them to control them or realise when something is deemed to be rude or inappropriate.

Anthropology Titbit The earliest known example of a highchair comes from the late seventeenth century. Later, Victorian highchairs often featured wheels, so the child could be wheeled in them from room to room.

Simply, if they are bored at the table and done with eating, they are going to let everybody know about it, whether you're at home or in a five-star restaurant. The best solution here (aside from not going to a five-star restaurant with a toddler in the first place) is to let them get down and run and play. Eventually, as their brain matures, they will begin to sit still and quietly for longer, they will start to understand social rules and, most importantly, they will learn to mimic the table manners that you yourself display. The toddler years are just not the time for this (yet) though.

Sleep development from two to three years

At this age, most toddlers are sleeping between ten and eleven hours at night, with the average sleep onset being at 8.30 p.m. and average wake time 7 a.m.[3] Night wakings are sadly still common, with 35 per cent of toddlers waking at least once a night, 24 per cent waking twice and 16 per cent waking three or more times.[4]

Research has found that toddlers who nap in the day sleep for less time at night, with longer daytime naps resulting in a shorter duration of night-time sleep.[5] This isn't necessarily a bad thing, though; if your toddler still naps in the daytime, and you – and they – are happy with their sleep at night, then there is no reason to lose, or shorten, their daytime nap. If your

> **Anthropology Titbit** Toddlers in Australia have an average bedtime of 7.30 p.m., but toddlers in Taiwan don't go to bed until 10 p.m.[6]

family is struggling with sleep at night, however, and your toddler does still nap in the daytime, you may want to consider shortening or dropping the daytime nap. Alternatively, if the daytime nap is still working for you, another option is to push

PARENTING Q&A

Q. *My toddler is always wide awake between 1 and 2 a.m. It doesn't matter whether they nap or not, or what time we do bedtime. Why is this?*

A. *Your toddler is exhibiting something known as polyphasic sleep. As a species, we all used to sleep like this until a couple of hundred years ago, splitting our night into two halves known as 'first sleep' and 'second sleep', with a period of waking in the middle. Your toddler's sleeping pattern is therefore normal – they just haven't learned yet that they were born in the twenty-first century where we sleep through the night. They will learn this in time, naturally, by observing your sleeping habits. Until this happens, the best way to discourage middle-of-the-night parties is to keep everything calm, quiet and dark at night. Don't leave their bedroom with them (for instance, going to your living area) and instead lie with them, reassure them and let them know that it's time to sleep.*

your toddler's bedtime back, so that they go to sleep later at night. The problem really only arises when parents and carers try to keep the daytime nap, but still expect their toddler to go to sleep early in the evening, sleep through the night and wake at a reasonable time in the morning.

One common sleep issue that parents and carers of toddlers encounter is the asynchrony between the time toddlers are put to bed at night and the innate body clock (circadian rhythm) and sleep needs of toddlers. Research from the University of Colorado has found that toddlers who are put to bed before their bodies have started to secrete a sufficient amount of the sleep hormone, melatonin, find it much harder to fall asleep than those whose bedtimes correlate with their melatonin levels.[7] The average time in the evening for melatonin onset for toddlers is 7.40, indicating that aiming for a sleep onset time of around 8 p.m. is biologically appropriate for them.

If you are aiming for sleep onset at around 8 p.m., a good bedtime routine for a two- to three-year-old might look like this:

7 p.m. – offer a small bedtime snack
7.15 p.m. – bath time
7.30 p.m. – into your toddler's bedroom for them to change into pyjamas
7.40 p.m. – bedtime story
7.45 p.m. – cuddles until they are asleep.

My aunt gave me the best advice: put her to sleep yourself every night. Sing to her and cradle her in your arms and sit by her side – every night, because one day you won't be able to.
Salma Hayek, actress

Moving to a bed from a cot

Most parents move their toddler out of their cot and into a
bed at some point between two and three years. Often, the
choice to make the move is dictated by a new baby arriv-
ing and the cot being needed for the newborn; sometimes
safety necessitates the move if the toddler has learned how
to climb out of the cot; sometimes the toddler outgrows
the cot; and sometimes the move is a choice made by
parents and carers in an attempt to improve their toddler's
sleep. Whatever the reason for the move, you should be
prepared for your toddler's sleep to be disturbed tempor-
arily while they get used to the change, but the following
tips can help to smooth the transition:

* Get your toddler involved in selecting their new bed.

* Don't change everything all at once. It may be
  tempting to redecorate at this time but leaving the
  old décor can help your toddler to feel more settled
  while they get used to the new bed.

* If you have space, set the bed up in the room for a
  while before you use it. If your toddler still naps, you
  could try for naps in the bed and bedtime at night
  still in the cot. If they don't nap, then spend time
  cuddling on the bed and sit on it together to read
  their bedtime story.

* Make sure everything in the room is baby-proofed;
  for instance, there are no dangling cords (from blinds
  and electrical equipment) and fix heavy furniture to
  the wall.

* If your toddler wanders out of bed in the night, just
  gently take them back and lie with them, cuddling,

until they go to sleep again. Don't chastise or punish them, or be tempted to use rewards (such as a sticker chart) to try to encourage them to stay in bed. Remember, their prefrontal cortex is very immature and they are unable to control their big feelings.

Instead of using a toddler bed, or a regular single/twin bed, you may instead consider setting up a Montessori floor bed for your toddler. This is a single mattress placed on the floor, with some slats underneath to create air flow. You can also get special floor bed frames, such as those in the shape of a house to make it more fun for your toddler. The beauty of the floor bed is it reduces the worry of your toddler falling out of bed accidentally, gives them more autonomy as getting in and out is easier and also allows you to lie next to them while they fall asleep and then easily sneak away.

PARENTING Q&A

Q. *Is there anything we can do to stop early-morning waking? My two-year-old is wide awake at 5.30 a.m. every day!*

A. *Unfortunately, early-morning waking is the human norm; it's actually we – as adults – who have problematic sleep when we sleep late after sunrise. However, if your little one still naps, this may be a sign that they are ready to drop their nap, or that they could do with a slightly later bedtime. Finally, check if there are any noises in your home that occur around 5.30 a.m. that could be causing your toddler to wake at the same time every day, such as your boiler clicking on.*

Social and psychological development from two to three years

When your toddler throws a cup of water from their high-chair, empties the contents of your purse or wallet, removes everything from a cupboard without permission (sometimes hiding things somewhere else or leaving them scattered all over the floor), drops their favourite toy into the toilet pan or hides the TV remote control under the sofa, they're not being naughty, despite what you may think. These are all common behaviours you would expect to see at this age. There is no naughty intention behind their actions – they are all wonderful examples of your toddler's natural curiosity and a desire to learn and discover.

Schemas

Children learn by experience. Or, more specifically, they learn when they reflect on something they do or did. We can tell them of our own experiences, and we can give them advice, but they only truly learn when they do or go through something themselves and especially when it is performed repeatedly. Understanding the repetitive patterns in the behaviour of young children, particularly during their play,

> Children think differently than adults . . .
> Children actively explore the world and environment
> around them. Therefore, they are little scientists on
> a voyage of observation and assimilation.
> *Jean Piaget, Swiss psychologist*

is important, especially when they are behaving in ways that could be deemed 'naughty'.

The word 'schemas' is used frequently among early-years education and childcare professionals to describe these repetitive actions, highlighting different patterns relating to specific behaviours:

Connection schema   In this schema, children learn how to connect things together. They will often be engrossed in building train tracks, sticking building blocks together or laying pieces of paper on the floor to make a path.

Containing schema   The containing schema occurs when children place objects into a container of some form. For instance, they may put all their crayons into an empty bag or inside a large box.

Enveloping schema   In this schema, children learn to cover things up. For example, they may cover their teddy bear with a blanket or their food with a napkin.

Positioning schema   Here, children are learning about the positions of one object in relation to another. They will often move their food around to different places on their plate or they may want to sit somewhere different from where they have been instructed.

Rotation schema   This is all about objects rotating. Children may be engrossed by the washing machine or the motion of wheels turning. They will often try to turn things that they think might rotate, such as the hands of a clock or a ball along the floor.

Trajectory schema   The trajectory schema teaches children about movement and direction. They will often throw items to observe their trajectories – food from their highchair, for example, or water thrown into the air.

Transforming schema Here, the child is interested in an object's changing properties. They may pour their juice into their porridge, for example, and explore the resulting transformation with their fingers. Or they may pour sand from their sand pit into their hair, to feel the change in texture.

Transporting schema This schema describes the action of children moving objects from one place to another. For instance, moving cans stacked in a cupboard to a different area of the kitchen or pushing a cart containing building blocks from one part of the garden to another.

Understandably, many of these schemas can be problematic for parents and carers. The child's learning is often at odds with social rules and expectations and can often be very messy. Parents and carers would much rather their children

Parent Observation 'My son was absolutely obsessed with the transporting schema for months. He was forever moving things around the house; it was like living with a poltergeist! I would put something down and then go to find it, only to find he had carried it off in his nursery bag and left it somewhere else. Once I realised what was happening I bought him a big car transporter toy – it was by far his favourite toy and he would play with it for hours, moving his toy cars around in it.'

Because children grow up, we think a child's purpose is to grow up. But a child's purpose is to be a child.
Tom Stoppard, British playwright and screenwriter

PARENTING Q&A

Q. *Is it possible for my toddler to be going through several schemas at once?*

A. *Yes, absolutely! You may find that your toddler shows signs of several schemas at a time, although there is usually one that it is their primary focus. Conversely, you may not notice signs of any schema-related play at all for a while. The patterns of schemas can be different for all children.*

didn't pour juice in their dinner, empty a packet of baby wipes and put them all into the toilet bowl or rearrange the contents of the kitchen cupboards, but they can rest assured that this behaviour is not only normal, but also indicative of great learning. And once you can spot the schema that your child is particularly interested in, you can encourage their learning with appropriate activities and schema-related toys.

Language and communication from two to three years

Your toddler's vocabulary will expand dramatically during this period, growing to around a thousand words by the time they turn three. They have a voracious appetite to learn, and the word you will probably hear most often during this period is 'Why?' Asking the names of different things is also a popular question, and while both can be irritating, it is helpful to remember that your toddler's curiosity is the best tool to aid their language development.

> **FUN FACT**
>
> *While it is true that boys often speak later than girls, researchers think this may have little to do with biology, and more with the fact that we speak more to baby and toddler girls. In other words, the later language development of most toddler boys may be due to societal factors and influences.*[8]

At two years old, children will be increasingly stringing two or three words together to form short sentences, and four or five by the time they turn three. Toddlers' speech is usually more understandable to others during this period (as opposed to just their parents and carers). Most will shorten longer words, saying 'yog' instead of 'yoghurt', for example, and may also stumble over those containing several different sounds. More complicated sounds, such as 'th' and 'ch', can take time to master, and you may find your toddler pronounces them incorrectly or with a slight lisp. This is usually outgrown as their language skills mature. Some stuttering and stammering remain normal at this age, as they struggle to verbalise all the ideas in their minds. Most children will naturally outgrow this

> **FUN FACT**
>
> *It may be tempting to use flashcards with your toddler to expand their vocabulary, but while they may learn the words from the flashcards and be able to recall and recite them with ease, this doesn't help with using them in their everyday language. Children need meaningful interactions with new words to learn them properly and flashcards don't provide these.*

There are many little ways to enlarge your child's world.
Love of books is the best of all.
Jacqueline Kennedy, former First Lady of the United States

within a few months; until they do, try to stay calm and quiet and listen patiently to them, rather than attempting to finish their sentences for them, or saying things like, 'Think about what you want to say.'

If you are worried about your toddler's speech for any reason, particularly if they are late to talk, then do consult your family doctor or health visitor, who may refer you to a speech therapist. You may be advised to 'wait and see' how your child's language develops, but early intervention leads to the best outcomes, so the sooner you speak to a professional about your concerns the better.

At this age, toddlers begin to understand nouns and pronouns and the difference between 'yours' and 'mine' (albeit everything tends to be 'mine' for them). Verbal comprehension continues to grow, including more complex instructions from carers, such as those containing two distinct steps, such as 'Go to the cupboard and get me your coat.' By the time they reach the age of three, most children understand plurals and the difference between 'car' and 'cars'.

Your toddler will now listen to, and understand, short stories (although getting them to sit still while you read to them is a whole other skill) and will remember elements of the stories, too. This means reading regularly with your toddler becomes more important than ever.

Play is our brains' favourite way of learning.
O. Fred Donaldson, American play specialist

Play ideas for two to three years

Play preferences for this age focus heavily on activities that embrace schemas. By understanding and embracing these preferences, you can create many ideas that will entertain your toddler for little outlay.

Connection schema   Create roads out of coloured pieces of paper or card laid on the floor for your toddler to drive a car over. Or use wooden building blocks laid out in a line to form a train track to push a train toy along.

Containing schema   Use an old bag for your toddler to pack their toys into or decorate a cardboard box with a lid to make an enclosed bed for their favourite cuddly toy.

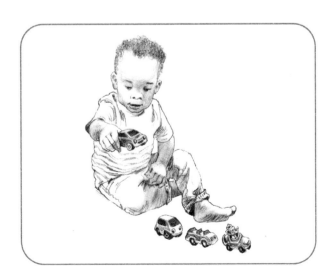

Enveloping schema   Make a duvet for your child's favourite teddy, using scraps of old material; or use a blanket to create a fort for them to hide in.

Rotation schema   Take the wheels off old broken toys and fix them onto a piece of wood or MDF sheet, for your toddler to spin; or use hooks, so that they can select the wheels to hang up themselves. They might also like to play with the hands of a wooden time-teaching clock.

Create a story sack for your toddler

Story sacks are cloth bags containing a favourite book, accompanied by objects and toys that appear in the story. For instance, if the book is *The Gruffalo*, the sack could also contain:

- a Gruffalo cuddly toy
- some wooden toy trees
- a pine cone
- a toy mouse
- a long, rubber snake
- an owl finger puppet
- a fox mask
- an acorn.

As you read through the story, you and your toddler can select the items that correspond with the words, role playing with them or using them like a matching game. Your toddler can even retell the story using just the objects. Story sacks are great for toddlers, combining their vivid imaginations, love of stories and the containing schema.

Trajectory schema   Get outside and encourage your toddler to throw a ball, beanbag or frisbee. In the summer, they may enjoy throwing water balloons with you and dodging the water.

Transforming schema   Mix cornflour and water (2 cups of cornflour to 1 cup of water) in a large plastic bowl to create something known as oobleck. Oobleck is fascinating for toddlers to play with – it feels wet and sticky when they plunge their fingers into it, but they come out dry and clean.

Recommended toys

The following are popular toys for two to three years:

- Wooden building blocks
- Wooden train sets
- Toy cars, trucks and transporters
- Baby dolls (especially great for toddlers who have welcomed a new baby sibling)
- Toy kitchen

Parent Observation   'My toddler's favourite toy is a toy hoover; he loves to copy me when I'm doing the housework, and his hoover goes everywhere with him.'

There are no seven wonders in the eyes of a child.
There are seven million.
Walt Streightiff, American author

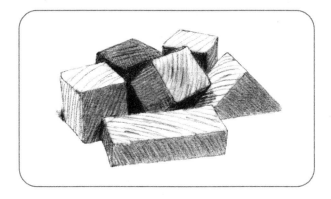

- Mud kitchen (for the garden)
- Stickle bricks
- Duplo blocks
- Threading buttons and chunky beads
- Puzzles
- Skittles sets
- Water-play toys

Raising a toddler can be hard, what with the non-stop 'Why?' questions, the big feelings and the tantrums, the defiance and constant cries of 'No!' and 'Me do it!' These can all feel frustrating and often draining for parents and carers, but as hard as it is to raise a toddler, it's much harder to *be* one. Understanding quite how amazing your little one's development is at this age and stopping to look through their eyes and view the world with wonder can help when it all gets a little too much. Remember, nothing your toddler does at this age is meant to deliberately annoy you. Their level of brain development simply doesn't allow them to be 'naughty'.

Let's move on now to the next year: the period between their third and fourth birthdays.

9

Three to Four Years

Your little one is now officially known as a preschooler. Although they are, of course, a child, officially they are not referred to as such until they turn five years old.

The preschooler years are all about your child's learning and the widening of their social circles. Whether they attend preschool or nursery, stay home with you or spend their days with a nanny or childminder, the emphasis of this year is on slowly branching out from their secure base with you and blossoming into a sociable and confident explorer, ready to take on the world and learn about everything in it.

How the brain develops from three to four years

This period is still very much about physical growth, new synaptic connections and pruning and continuing myelination. The areas of the brain responsible for conscious movement control and emotions are by now well connected, meaning that your three-year-old is proficient at gross motor skills

Neuroscience Nugget A preschooler's brain is around 80 per cent of its fully grown adult size and uses a whopping 30 per cent of all the body's nutrition each day.

Neuroscience Nugget By the time a child turns three, 80 per cent of the synaptic connections in their brain are already formed. These connections amount to around a thousand trillion in number!

and mastering an increasing number of fine motor ones. As well as this maturing physical control, they will continue to experience many big emotions, thanks to development in their limbic system. What they still don't have at this age, however, is a well-connected prefrontal cortex. This means that for all their physical skills and dexterity and their capacity to feel a whole spectrum of emotions, they still don't possess the ability to control these things when life gets overwhelming (which happens often).

Having said that, this doesn't mean that nothing is happening with the prefrontal cortex. The development trajectory of this area of the brain is not linear, and although vast changes occur in the prefrontal cortex in the first three years of life, directed largely by the experiences a child has during this period, research has shown that peak synaptic density here is achieved significantly later than in other areas of the brain. So while rapid change occurs in the area during infancy and toddlerhood, the process of synaptic development and pruning occurs later, meaning that the refinement of the area happens much slower than it does elsewhere in the brain.[1]

What does this mean for parents and carers? Well, firstly, we should reset our expectations of preschoolers and understand that many of the behaviours so frequently disciplined (such as tantrums, whining, a lack of impulse control and so-called antisocial behaviour, like biting, hitting and kicking) are simply indicative of a developmentally immature

> Child development does not mean developing your child
> into the person you think they should be but helping
> them develop into the best person they are meant to be.
> *Toni Sorenson, author*

prefrontal cortex. Secondly, we should understand that both the way we treat children at this age and the experiences they have will directly impact the way their brains develop. This is a critical and sensitive period for the prefrontal cortex and, as such, the role of a parent or carer is to protect and nurture its growth, through empathetic, compassionate and supportive care.

Research following children from preschool through to age nine shows that those who received more nurturing care during their early years had a more developed hippocampus than those who received less.[2] Hippocampal volume is important because it impacts memory, learning and the ability to retain what is learned and to focus during learning.

Physical development from three to four years

Physically, your preschooler will start to look very different during this period – not just because they are growing in height, but also because their body-fat percentage starts to decrease, while increasing muscle tone means that their typical toddler shape of a curved back and sticking-out tummy turns to more of an upright adult posture. This all makes them look significantly leaner and much more grown up, and far from just changing their appearance, it also means that your preschooler is much more skilled at physical movements now.

Physical milestones

Between the ages of three and four, your preschooler will likely master many gross motor skills, including:

- running around different obstacles, keeping their balance while doing so
- standing on one foot for several seconds
- hopping from one foot to another, and perhaps on one foot for a few seconds
- walking up and down stairs without needing to hold your hand
- climbing – onto play equipment and furniture
- riding a scooter, a balance bike or bicycle with stabilisers
- following a straight line marked on the floor, keeping their balance
- walking with a 'heel-toe' pattern (putting their heels down before their toes, rather than favouring tiptoes, as they may have done in the toddler years).

Fine motor skills are also rapidly developing, and by the end of this period your preschooler will likely be able to:

- tackle larger buttons (both undoing and doing them up)

Children more than ever need opportunities to be in their bodies in the world. Jumping rope, bicycling, stream hopping and fort building. It's this engagement between limbs of the body and bones of the earth where true balance and centredness emerge.
David Sobel, American environmental educationalist

Art is a place for children to learn to trust their ideas,
themselves, and to explore what is possible.
MaryAnn F. Kohl, author and educator

- pull zips up and down (with help to get them started)
- cut into a sheet of paper
- stack between eight and ten wooden blocks on top of each other
- build towers and other structures with Duplo-type play bricks
- open and close a lunchbox
- complete a jigsaw puzzle with four to eight pieces.

When it comes to mark making, by the end of this period, your preschooler will move to holding a pencil with a tripod grasp

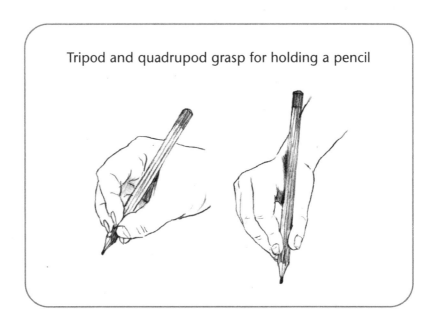

Tripod and quadrupod grasp for holding a pencil

(using their thumb and their middle and index fingers) or a quadrupod grasp (using their thumb and their middle, index and ring fingers).

Your preschooler's drawings will now likely include the following rough shapes:

- Circles
- Squares
- Dots
- Crossing lines, often imitating the letters T and H

This is also the age at which children can start to draw images of people, usually featuring a large head drawn straight onto a very long pair of legs with shorter arms, omitting the body entirely. Drawing is very much done with intention at this age, and if asked to explain their work, preschoolers will likely be able to describe the pictures and the stories behind them, even if you find it hard to interpret them.

Typical drawing skills for three- to four-year-olds

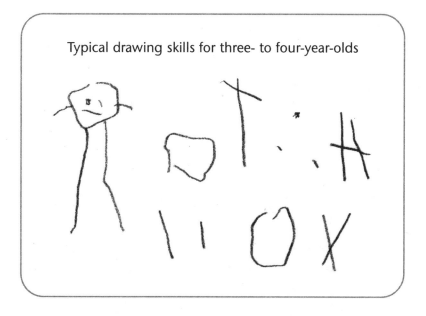

Feeding and eating from three to four years

As your preschooler grows and is exposed to food in different settings (such as at nursery and birthday parties), as well as understanding and falling prey to advertising and marketing in supermarkets, they will probably ask you for more palatable foods and snacks, like chocolate, sweets and crisps. It may be tempting to entirely restrict these 'junk foods' or keep them for special occasions only, but a more mindful approach (and indeed, one that has been shown to have the best outcomes in the long term) is to allow children to self-regulate these foods.

The language used by adults to label palatable foods as 'treats', 'sometimes foods', 'unhealthy' or similar can make a child more likely to crave them as they get older. When we give food this sort of status it greatly impacts on how we interact with it. Removing this sort of language from discussion of food is the healthiest approach – so instead of calling a cake a 'treat', simply call it 'food' or just 'cake'.

Restricting palatable foods (think crisps, chocolate and the like) is also shown consistently to be a large risk factor in children being unable to self-regulate later in life as they grow and gain independence surrounding what they can eat and when. This often results in overeating and bingeing on previously forbidden items in the teen and young adult years, which can and does impact weight gain.

Anthropology Titbit Ketchup is a universal favourite among preschoolers due to its sweet taste, with Swedish preschoolers eating more of it than any other children in the world.

Why you should let your preschooler play with their food

While many parents and carers try to stop their preschooler playing with their food and focus on the use of cutlery and observing table manners, research shows that allowing and, indeed, encouraging them to play with their food improves their eating – particularly when it comes to trying and liking vegetables.[3] Just like babies, preschoolers still learn about the world best – including what they eat – when the experience is as multi-sensory as possible. If they are allowed to touch their food, and play with it, this helps them to learn about and familiarise themselves with it, thus reducing neophobia and increasing acceptance. So the next time your preschooler sticks their hands in their soup, try to hold back on telling them to use their spoon, swooping in with a cloth to wipe them up, and instead, reassure yourself that they are learning to be a better eater.

Research shows that children learn to self-regulate their food intake if adults don't interfere based on their own learned beliefs and disordered eating behaviours.[4] While they may eat several sweets or cakes in a short span of time, preschoolers will tend to eat 'healthily' if you look at their food intake over

FUN FACT
Preschoolers who watch their parents repeatedly eating vegetables at mealtimes are more likely to try – and like – the same vegetable.

a whole day, or week, rather than focusing on what they are eating in a short time span. This doesn't mean giving them entirely free rein over their diets, but rather, allowing them to control *when* they eat items that you have already purchased. You may buy a multipack of seven chocolate bars in your weekly shop, for example, and rather than restricting them to 'only one per day' or 'only after you have eaten your dinner', you allow them the choice of eating earlier in the day, or eating two or three at once, leaving them with none for other days. By giving your preschooler autonomy over food when they are younger, you will be giving them the best chance to learn how to self-regulate their eating around palatable foods as they grow – a skill that many adults have yet to master.

Sleep development from three to four years

By now, your preschooler is likely to be sleeping for longer periods at night, with far fewer night wakings. They will still wake and need you at night sometimes, though, especially when they have nightmares, need to go to the toilet or want comforting when they are anxious or ill.

Most children of this age will get between ten and thirteen hours' sleep in a twenty-four-hour period, and almost all of

Anthropology Titbit Preschoolers in India tend to have much later bedtimes than their European and American counterparts. The average bedtime for a preschooler in India is 10.26 p.m., but Indian children usually still nap in the daytime, whereas those in Western countries who have earlier bedtimes usually do not.[5]

this is at night, as most children will drop their nap during this period, if they have not already done so.

Night terrors and nightmares

Nightmares are common at this age, with at least 50 per cent of preschoolers regularly having them and needing their parents' help to get back to sleep after waking from one. Night terrors, in contrast, are rarer, affecting between 1 and 6 per cent of preschoolers.

Night terrors are a parasomnia – an unusual behavioural and physiological phenomenon that occurs during sleep. Unlike nightmares, they happen in a stage of deep sleep called non-REM, categorised by the absence of dreams. Nightmares, on the other hand, happen in REM sleep and often the child wakes up and retains a memory of them.

Common symptoms of night terrors include:

- thrashing around during sleep
- lashing out, biting and hitting
- screaming
- shouting
- eyes opening with a non-focused, 'glazed' look
- remaining deeply asleep and being extremely difficult to wake
- having no recollection of the event upon waking.

Night terrors are most usual between the ages of three and eight, although they can happen earlier and later (approximately 4 per cent of adults still experience them at some point). They also affect boys more than girls, whereas nightmares affect both equally. Terrors usually occur in the earlier part of the night, before midnight, whereas nightmares tend to occur in the later, often up until the morning.

One of the most important things to understand about night terrors is that due to the deep sleep state the child is in, you shouldn't try to wake them. Instead, you should focus your energy on keeping them as safe as possible. Make sure that they cannot knock anything onto themselves or fall, causing injury. Once you have ensured that your child is safe, the best thing you can do is to stay in the room until the terror passes. Keep the lights low and remind yourself that while difficult and highly stressful for you to watch, these episodes are not at all harmful and your child will not remember them in the morning.

Two specific things that have shown promise in scientific research regarding night terrors are scheduled awakening and omega-3 supplementation.

1. **Scheduled awakening** If night terrors are recurring, keep a diary of the times at which they happen. If there is a pattern, try to wake your child ten minutes before the episodes usually take place and keep them awake for five to ten minutes. This can disrupt their sleep cycle enough to stand a good chance of preventing the terrors.[6]

2. **Omega-3 supplementation** Supplementing with 600mg of omega-3 for a period of four months has been found to reduce the incidence of parasomnias. In addition, supplementation has also been shown to improve general sleep quantity in children.[7]

Good sleep hygiene is also important: ensure your child's bedroom is not too hot or too cold (18°C is ideal) and that they are comfortable and not overtired. Reduce stress as much as possible, make sure the child's diet is healthy and be mindful of lighting. Unfortunately, however, aside from scheduled awakening and omega-3 supplementation, there is no scientific evidence in support of any other treatments. In most cases, it

PARENTING Q&A

Q. *When should you take away nappies at night? My three-and-a-half-year-old has been dry in the daytime for almost a year, but there is no sign of dropping the night nappy yet.*

A. *Night dryness is developmental and is based upon the secretion of something known as antidiuretic hormone (ADH). Most children will secrete enough ADH to go without nappies at night around the time of their fourth birthday, although 10 per cent still need them at the age of six, and it is not considered problematic until the child's seventh birthday.*

is simply a case of waiting for the child to outgrow the night terrors and keeping them safe while they are happening.

Social and psychological development from three to four years

The preschool years often herald the arrival of friendships, and you may find your child starts to form a close bond with one or two children of a similar age. At this age, children begin to understand the concept of friendship and will often name children that they are friends with when asked 'Who is your friend?' or 'Who are your friends?' Friendship can be tricky at this age, however, as preschoolers struggle with social rules, and their underdeveloped sense of empathy, difficulty sharing and controlling their impulses (including lashing out at others when they are feeling stressed) can often cause fractious relationships. Of course, we know that these aren't signs of naughtiness or antisocial behaviour – they are typical of all preschoolers with immature brains. The best way to help your preschooler with forming friendships is to role model empathy and turn taking at home with them and to discuss the idea of friendships and how to make friends with others, perhaps with the help of some appropriate children's books.

Theory of mind: why preschoolers are egocentric

Preschoolers are naturally egocentric – in other words, they think only of themselves, with little regard for the thoughts and feelings of others. Although this would be a negative trait in adults, in preschoolers it is developmentally normal. The ability of a child to understand the viewpoint of others, and the underpinning of them having empathy for them, is commonly referred to as 'theory of mind'. Theory of mind explains how children (and adults) appreciate that we are all individuals with our own thoughts, beliefs and feelings and that these psychological states will differ as we each have a unique experience of life.

Psychologists have long questioned the age at which theory of mind takes root, with the current view being that it begins in infancy, but there is a marked difference in development between three- and four-year-olds. Whereas most three-year-olds struggle with the idea that others have different thoughts, feelings and experiences to them, four-year-olds show a marked increase in understanding the individual thoughts and experiences of others and that they can be different to their own. In particular, research has shown that three-year-olds grapple with something known as 'false belief' – the ability to understand that others may believe something that is not true.[8] A good example of a false-belief test uses a sweet or chocolate box to disguise unexpected contents – for example, a chocolate box containing a paper clip. A three-year-old is shown the box and then the unexpected contents. They are asked, 'What do you think your mummy or daddy (who were not in the room when the child was shown the paper clip) will say is in this box?' In most cases, the three-year-old will answer 'a paper clip'. Of course, the correct answer would be that the parent will say the box contains sweets/chocolate – and that is the answer that children will mostly give once they are four years old, indicating that the development of false belief occurs somewhere around a child's fourth birthday. Why not give the experiment a try with your own child and see what they say?

How does this impact parents and carers of preschoolers? Being armed with an understanding of the acquisition of theory of mind can help them to reset their social expect-ations, particularly those involving empathy for others, such as willingness to share a toy – or rather *un*willingness to share, which is more developmentally appropriate for a three-year-old who is struggling with immature theory of mind.

PARENTING Q&A

Q. *Why does my child laugh when I tell them off?*

A. *Most preschoolers laugh when they are told off because of fear or stress. Rather than being a sign of defiance or rudeness, laughter in this situation is usually an indication of nervousness. It may also be caused by your preschooler misinterpreting your emotions due to a lack of theory of mind – because they do not understand that you may be angered by something that they find funny.*

Impulse control in the preschooler years

Although your preschooler's prefrontal cortex is more developed than it was during the toddler years, it is still far from mature. Therefore, impulse control is something they will inevitably struggle with, and no matter how many times you ask them not to touch something, for example, if their overriding impulse is to touch it, then that will always win out over any desire to please you. Again, this doesn't mean that your preschooler is being 'naughty' – they are doing the

The Stanford marshmallow test

In the 1970s, Stanford University professor of psychology Walter Mischel and student Ebbe Ebbesen devised a simple experiment looking at preschoolers' lack of impulse control and their innate drive towards instant gratification.[9]

Mischel and Ebbesen offered children a treat of either a pretzel or a marshmallow to choose from. Both the marshmallow and pretzel were left in view of the children, and they were told that the experimenter had to leave the room for a little while (the goal was fifteen minutes), and that if they waited, they would be allowed to eat their chosen treat when the experimenter returned. The children were also told that they could call out for the experimenter to return to the room earlier than planned, but if they called for them, they would receive their second-choice treat, not the first.

Another group of children were not given any instructions to wait for the experimenter, but were simply left with the treats when the experimenter left the room. A final group were either given a slinky toy to play with when the experimenter left the room or they were advised to think of something fun to do, such as sing a song, while they were alone to pass the time.

Mischel and Ebbesen found that the children who had been offered a reward (their desired treat) waited significantly longer before eating the treat (although most did not reach the specified fifteen minutes) than those who were not given any specific instructions. The children who were given a distraction to play with also waited significantly longer than those who had no distraction or treat on offer.

The results of this experiment give parents and carers of preschoolers two useful pieces of information. Firstly, if preschoolers are given something fun to distract them, or a novel toy to play with, it helps to improve their impulse control. Secondly, if preschoolers are given autonomy and are allowed to make a choice around receiving a desired treat, this can also help their impulse control in the short term. Both these findings can help in the real world when we need short-term compliance from our children.

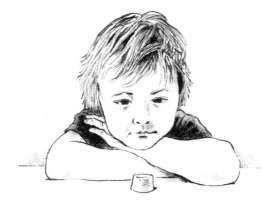

> The best way to make children good is to
> make them happy.
> *Oscar Wilde, Irish poet and playwright*

best they can with an immature brain. Impulse control will develop naturally in time, as their prefrontal cortex continues to mature; until then, the best way to encourage it is to model it yourself, while resetting your expectations of your child's behaviour. There is no point in punishing or scolding them for a behaviour that is beyond their years.

Language and communication from three to four years

Your preschooler welcomes their third birthday with a vocabulary of around a thousand words, but by the time they turn four, this has almost doubled. And it's not just their vocabulary that is growing; preschoolers begin to link more and more words together, forming short sentences of up to five words. Grammatically, speech matures further, too, with the use of plurals and adjectives, for example.

During this period, your preschooler begins to convey more complex ideas and to describe people and things with increasing accuracy. Children of this age utilise their language skills to learn more about the world around them, with frequent 'Why?' and 'How?' questions. As frustrating as the constant stream of questions can be, it is important to remember that everything is new in the eyes of a curious three-year-old and the world holds wonder and intrigue for them that we, as adults, have long since grown tired of. The best way to handle

> **Parent Observation** 'My daughter must have said the word 'why' about a hundred times every day from the age of three to four. It was infuriating and tiring, especially when we didn't know the answers to her questions, but if we didn't know the answers, we used it as a teaching opportunity when we tried to research the answer together. Looking back now, these are some of my fondest memories of this age, even though I hated them at the time!'

the constant questioning is to remind yourself of this and try to answer as accurately as possible and in a way that validates and makes them feel heard.

Technoference – how today's technology harms language development

Scientists researching the impact of the increasing use of technology on child development frequently warn of something known as technoference. This term is used to describe the harmful effects of parents and carers who are distracted by their phones, tablets, PCs and laptops when caring for young children. Research has found that the parents of children with language delay spend significantly more time on their mobile phones when they are with their children. Previous research has also highlighted the negative impact on parental responsivity towards children when an adult engages in screen time in the presence of their children.[10] This doesn't just negatively impact children's language development, but also their behaviour, with a correlation evident between children's difficult conduct and the time parents or carers spent using screen-based technology when caring for them.

When children spend more time on screens themselves this too can, and does, have a negative effect on their speech. Recent research has found that young children who spend more time playing on a tablet are more likely to develop language delay than their peers who have less screen time.[11]

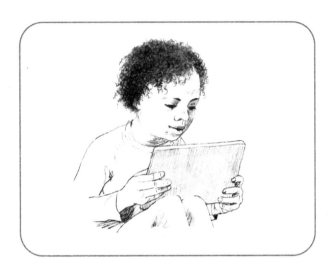

PARENTING Q&A

Q. *Is there a way that we can incorporate screen time into our three-year-old's day and reduce any bad effects?*

A. *The American Academy of Pediatrics recommends that children between three to five years of age should be restricted to a maximum of one hour of screen time per day. In addition to restricting the screen time itself, working to reduce passive watching has a protective effect. Try to engage with your toddler while they are using screens; for instance, commenting on what they are seeing and asking questions to encourage conversation.*

Play ideas for three to four years

Have you ever stopped to observe your three-year-old when they are playing in the presence of other children? It is likely that they are engaged in something known as 'parallel play'. Parallel play occurs when young children, usually between the ages of two and three and a half, play alongside each other, each engrossed in their own world and play. While their physical proximity may indicate to adults that they are playing together, most younger preschoolers will play alone, although, as they get older, they will increasingly pay attention to their neighbours. Parallel play and the careful watching of their close-by peers helps preschoolers to learn how to socialise and, eventually, to form friendships as their solitary play morphs into playing together. This next stage of play – where preschoolers show more interest in the play of their peers – is known as associative play and is usually observed between the ages of three and four. (**Note**: there are natural overlaps in the transition between play stages.) Finally, associative play gives way to co-operative play – usually after the child's fourth birthday, when they are fully engaged in play with their peers.

Why fewer toys are better

It can be tempting to splurge on the newest toy you've seen advertised and think your preschooler will enjoy, but toys are one area of childhood where less is definitely more: the more children have, the more likely they are to complain of boredom.

As children grow, the overprovision of toys can stifle their imaginations. Research has found that removing toys from children results in them becoming not only more creative, but more social, too. In an experiment entitled '*Der Spielzeugfreie Kindergarten*' ('The Nursery Without Toys'), all toys were removed from children at a nursery for a period of three months, the only items left being chairs and blankets.[12] Initially, the researchers found that the children were bored, but they quickly readjusted and were soon building dens and enjoying their new set-up. By the end of the experimental period, not only were the children playing imaginatively and creatively, but they were also more confident and social with each other displaying better interpersonal relationships and less friction and fighting. This led the researchers to claim that children can be 'suffocated' by the presence of toys and also find it harder to concentrate when surrounded by them.

What can this research tell us as parents and carers? Firstly, it's a good idea to thin out the toy supply, removing ones that are barely or rarely played with to encourage better play and more imagination. Next is the idea of rotating toys. When at the end of the experiment, toys were reintroduced to the nursery, the children were happy to see them return. So the saying 'absence makes the heart grow fonder' applies to toys, too, and it's a good idea to put some away in a cupboard for a month or two to make them fresh and give them novelty value. Finally, never underestimate the play value in simple everyday objects. In the case of the experiment, it was some chairs and blankets, but there are many other options, such

Play is often talked about as if it were a relief from serious learning. But for children play is serious learning. Play is really the work of childhood.
Fred Rogers, American TV host

as creating houses or spaceships from old cardboard boxes, using mud to 'bake' pies or create models or even putting an old sheet of bubble-wrap packaging on the floor to jump on. Don't be constrained by the label 'toy' when everyday items can bring as much joy – if not more.

Recommended toys

Following on from the previous point, that less is more when it comes to toys, choosing them carefully for your preschooler is important, to get the most value, both in terms of play and outlay. These are some of the most popular toys for this age range:

- Duplo and Lego bricks
- Wooden train sets
- Toy cars, trucks and transporters
- Real-world play (for instance, a play supermarket or post office)
- A doll's house and figures
- Jigsaw puzzles with twenty-four medium-sized pieces
- A climbing frame or garden swing if you have outdoor space
- A Pikler triangle or wooden climbing frame, for indoors
- Model-making equipment, such as play dough or kinetic sand
- A first bike or a scooter
- A first paint set

Note: many of these are the same toys as for two- to three-year-olds. Classic toy choices can last for many years.

*

You will always be your child's favourite toy.
Vicki Lansky, American author

The preschooler period is when children blossom into truly sociable beings, and watching them engaged in play with their peers, as they chat away, is heartwarming. You are still the centre of your child's world, though, and while their orbit is ever increasing, it is always you they will return to when they need to feel safe and secure – a testament to the love and nurturing you have given them. It is this attachment and sense of security that will see them on their way even further once they turn four and enter the school years, which is the subject of the next – and final – chapter.

10

Four to Five Years

The year between your child's fourth and fifth birthdays is all about thoughts of choosing and starting school and looking forward to a bright future, full of new learning and possibilities. It is also a time to look back at the remarkable growth and development they have achieved so far, thanks to your loving care and dedication. Their personality really blossoms at this age, and they begin to form closer bonds and friendships as they socialise more and more with their peers. This is an exciting time indeed, for parents and carers and children alike.

How the brain develops from four to five years

Between the ages of four and five, a child's brain still has a way to go, although some areas are more developed than others. The part of the brain responsible for movement and motor control (the motor cortex, situated in the frontal lobe) is the most mature at this age, and it is the first area in which

Enjoy the little things, for one day you may look back
and realise they were the big things.
Robert Brault, American author

Neuroscience Nugget By the time a child is five years old, their brain has reached 90 per cent of its final adult size.

myelination is completed, meaning that synaptic impulses are well insulated and thus as fast and effective as possible.[1]

The prefrontal cortex is continuing to form new synaptic connections at this age, as well as myelinating existing, re-inforced ones. This ongoing development of the area of the brain (responsible for higher cognitive functions, such as the ability to evaluate a situation and weigh up a decision or action, to adapt behaviour flexibly based upon experience and to organise and control actions and thoughts) will not be complete until the child is in their twenties. Many of the behaviours that parents and carers hope to see their children exhibiting at this age are controlled by the prefrontal cortex, and no amount of discipline will help them to behave in a mature way while it is still developing.

During this period, brain development continues to be 'experience-dependent', meaning that new connections form because of new things that occur during the child's life. Sci-entists once believed the brain to be unchangeable once it has finished developing, but we now know that it has a great

Every child has an inner timetable for growth – a pattern unique to him. Growth is not steady, forward, upward progression. It is instead a switchback trail; three steps forward, two back, one around the bushes and a few simply standing before another forward leap.
Dorothy Corkille Briggs, American author and educator

How to encourage your four-year-old's brain development

Research has found that the more mental stimulation children get at four years old, the better developed the areas of their brain responsible for language and cognition will be when they are teenagers.[2]

Researchers studied brain scans of four-year-olds, then scanned the same children again between seventeen and nineteen years old to compare the changes. They also took comprehensive notes on the children's home lives and activities, including the number of books at their disposal, whether they had access to and played musical instruments and whether their toys were designed to help them learn about things such as shapes and colours. Analysis of brain scans in the late teens was linked to the children's brain development at age four, as well as to the level of cognitive stimulation they received in early childhood.

What can parents and carers take from this research? Quite simply that stimulating your four-year-old with lots of books, music and carefully chosen play activities can have a long-lasting positive impact on their brain development.

degree of 'neural plasticity', meaning that it can change and adapt to new occurrences throughout life, with neurogenesis (the creation of new neurons) and synaptogenesis (the creation of new synapses) continuing well into adulthood (albeit nowhere near the exuberant pace observed during infancy).

Neural pruning also continues during this age, with connections that are rarely used being removed, so as to focus on more important, regularly strengthened ones. Pruning in

PARENTING Q&A

Q. *I have heard that difficult behaviour from four-year-olds is due to something called a 'limbic leap'. Is this true?*

A. *Sadly, not. While it would be nice to package children's brain development up into an easy-to-understand series of predictable 'leaps', this is simply not how it works. The limbic system (the part of the brain responsible for feeling big emotions) is already well matured by the time a child is four years old and there is no big leap at this age; rather, there is a continuous change in synaptic development, myelination and neural pruning.*

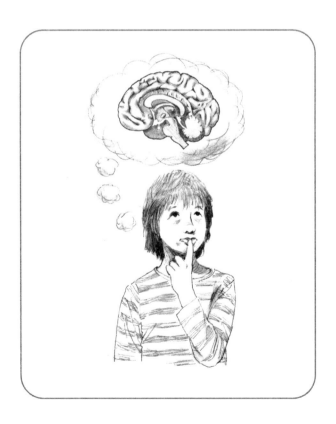

the visual cortex of the brain (responsible for sight and the processing of visual information) is complete at some time between the child's fourth and sixth birthdays; in contrast, areas related to higher cognitive functioning continue to be pruned all the way through the teen years and into the twenties.[3]

Physical development from four to five years

By the time they are four years old, children have mastered a huge number of gross motor skills, including running, jumping, hopping, climbing and balancing. Their fine motor skills are also maturing at a fast rate.

At this age, children need plenty of opportunities to move their bodies freely; four-year-olds aren't meant to sit still and

> We spend the first year of a child's life teaching it to walk and talk and the rest of its life teaching it to shut up and sit down. There's something wrong there.
> *Neil deGrasse Tyson, American astrophysicist*

Parent Observation 'My little boy became obsessed with cutting everything when he was four. The best thing we ever bought was a special child-safe knife that he could use to help us prepare vegetables for dinner. He was so proud of helping to cook by cutting things up for us and it had a lovely knock-on effect of making him more likely to eat whatever he had cut up, too.'

quietly – they are meant to move and be loud! This is important to remember as they approach school-starting age and new behavioural expectations are placed upon them. Parents and carers can help children to adjust to the transition to school by providing plenty of opportunities for freedom of movement at home.

Physical milestones

Between your child's fourth and fifth birthdays, they will likely learn how to:

- balance on one foot
- dress and undress themselves independently (with help with fiddly buttons and zips)
- kick and throw a ball with a fairly accurate aim
- skip, with a rope
- jump backwards
- hop.

From a fine motor-skill development point of view, they will likely learn how to:

- tie their shoelaces
- cut in a straight line with scissors
- trace a line on a piece of paper with a pencil, to draw a letter or shape
- show consistent right- or left-handedness
- build or link a large tower or row of bricks, or small blocks (such as Lego)
- use a knife to cut their own soft food.

Mark making between four and five years

You will likely see a huge change in your child's mark-making skills as the year progresses, with their drawings becoming more purposeful and recognisable to you and others. You will see conscious patterns and they will be able to explain their picture to you, naming certain parts, such as animals or people.

Your four-year-old will experiment with more shapes in their drawing, including squares, circles, rectangles and sometimes triangles (although these are harder to draw than other shapes). When it comes to drawing people, four-year-olds progress from tadpole-like figures with large heads on long legs, to including a body, arms, fingers and facial features, such as eyes and a mouth. They may begin to draw hair and clothing, too, as they approach the age of five.

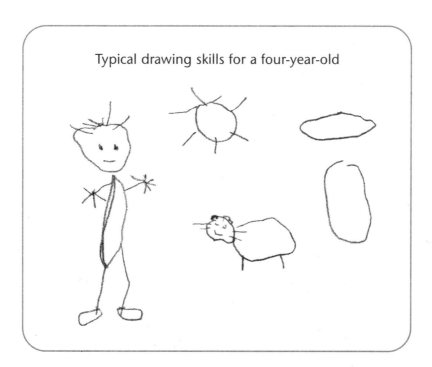

Typical drawing skills for a four-year-old

Anthropology Titbit In Sweden, children do not start formal schooling or learn to read and write until they are seven years old, before which they attend preschool where the emphasis is on play. Despite this, by the time they are ten years old, Swedish children have better literacy skills than most other European children who begin formal education much earlier.

A four-year-old will also attempt to trace a shape or letter – either that you have written or ones that appear in early handwriting books – and they may try to form letters themselves, especially those that appear in their name.

When it comes to holding a pencil or crayon, most children at this stage will use a 'dynamic tripod grasp', similar to that of an adult.

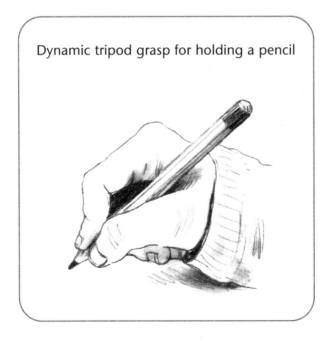

Dynamic tripod grasp for holding a pencil

A note on non-neurotypical development

As mentioned right at the start of this book, milestones are unique for each child. Some children will hit them early and some will hit them late, because all children are different. And many who are neurodivergent – those whose neurological development differs from the norm – will meet milestones at a different time.

If you notice that your child's development is not in line with the examples in this book, it may be that they are neurodivergent or have a special educational need (SEND), such as autism or ADHD (attention deficit hyperactivity disorder). If you are concerned, or you instinctively feel that their developmental curve is different from that which may be expected for their age, speak to your health visitor, family doctor or school SENCo (special educational needs co-ordinator), who can refer you for specialist diagnosis and support. (See also Resources, page 258, for support organisations.)

Feeding and eating from four to five years

While your four-year-old is now a much more independent eater, able to use a knife to cut their own food and an open-top cup with ease, the picky eating they experienced in the toddler and preschooler years can still be evident. Research has found that one in five children continues to be a fussy eater until they approach their teenage years,[4] with periods of picky eating lasting for at least two years in 40 per cent of children affected. As with picky and fussy eating in the earlier years,

FUN FACT
The average four-year-old needs to consume around 1200–1400 calories per day.

there is no quick-fix solution; rather, a mindful approach centred on understanding, patience and good role modelling is the best answer.

The benefits of involving children in the kitchen

Involving children with preparing family meals and baking is a wonderful way to spend time with them. Teaching them how to cook has many benefits, including the following:

Increasing self-esteem Teaching a child to make food from scratch can help their confidence, by creating a sense of ownership and pride.

A reduction in picky and fussy eating Research shows that children who are regularly involved in the preparation and cooking of vegetables are more likely to eat them.[5]

A reduction in obesity levels in adulthood Teaching children how to make healthy and nutritious meals gives them the skills they need to eat well as they grow.

Improvement in fine motor skills The various activities involved in cooking, such as chopping, kneading, rolling, pouring and stirring, are all brilliant for developing a child's fine motor skills.

Improved maths ability Cooking includes a lot of organic mathematics skills, such as weighing and measuring ingredients and calculating how much to buy when following a recipe.

Improved problem-solving skills and scientific understanding Children learn how to solve unexpected problems that may arise when cooking, such as understanding why a cake doesn't rise, why the broccoli boils dry on the hob or why a sauce turns out too runny.

Enhanced literacy and communication skills When you discuss a recipe and cooking instructions with your child and talk about the processes involved, it helps to expand their vocabulary; similarly, following a recipe from a book or online is a great way to prompt reading skills.

Understanding the environment When you cook regularly with children, it can lead naturally to conversations about sustainability and environmental issues – for instance, talking about buying locally grown produce and in-season fruits and vegetables.

Cooking with your four-year-old isn't just about the benefits for them, though. The time you spend connecting with them, giving them your undivided attention while in the kitchen, can have a fantastic impact on your bond with them. Plus, children who feel more connected to their parents or carers tend to behave better because their need for attention is being met, making day-to-day discipline easier.

> Cooking with kids is not just about ingredients, recipes and cooking. It's about harnessing imagination, empowerment and creativity.
> *Guy Fieri, American restaurateur, author and TV presenter*

Helping your four-year-old with school lunches

When your child starts school, they will need to navigate a whole new eating experience. If they will be taking packed lunches, make sure that you select a lunch box or bag that they can open independently, and one that can be easily recognised in a sea of thirty others. Also, be mindful of the contents of their lunch and their ability to handle packaging independently. For instance, squeezable yoghurt pouches seem appealing for young children, but they can often be difficult for little hands to open; a banana or satsuma may seem like a perfect snack, but peeling them unassisted can be tricky. While there will be midday staff supervising school lunchtimes, they are not able to look after all children, and if your child cannot eat their packed lunch without help, they may well come home with it uneaten at the end of the day.

If your child will be having school dinners, try to get hold of the menu in advance (they usually work on a two- or four-weekly rota) and go through any unknown dishes with them, so they know what to expect. You could make some of these at home in advance, so they are more familiar if you have a fussy eater. Finally, practise carrying their own plate or tray with them, as this is something they will have to do at school (but often not something they do at home).

Whatever your child eats for lunch at school, be prepared for them to be famished when you pick them up at the end of the day. Introducing an after-school snack as soon as they get home is a good idea (after-school daycare clubs all tend to offer one), as a child who is hangry (hungry/angry) will tend to have more tantrums than one who isn't. Breakfast-type food is a good option here.

Sleep development from four to five years

Between the ages of four and five, it is recommended that children get between ten and thirteen hours sleep within a twenty-four-hour period. Remember, sleep needs are individual, and while one child may need the full thirteen hours, others may be happy with only ten, or even nine. The average bedtime (sleep onset time) for a four-year-old is around 8–8.30 p.m., with an average wake time of around 7 a.m. Some children may wake earlier (waking at 5.30 or 6 a.m. isn't unusual at this age), which isn't a problem, so long as they are getting sufficient sleep.

Nightmares remain common at this age, with night terrors usually lessening a little as children get older. Night waking is often centred around nightmares and separation anxiety (this often reappears when children start school), so making sure your child feels as secure and as safe as possible is the key to better sleep in most cases.

How to improve your four-year-old's sleep

If sleep is still difficult, consider the following:

Make time for reconnecting before bedtime This is especially important for children who have been separated from their parents or carers during the day (because of school, for instance). Perhaps the best way to reconnect at this age is joining in with playtime together. Evenings in a family home are

Anthropology Titbit While the average bedtime for children in the UK is 7.55 p.m., in Hong Kong it is 10.17 p.m.

often rushed, with little time for play. We rush from activity to activity to dinner and then straight off to bed. Making time to actively play together as a family for half an hour (or as long as you can) before the bedtime routine begins can have a dramatically positive effect on sleep for most families.

Follow a consistent bedtime routine   Bedtime routines often slip as children get older and parents and carers believe they are no longer necessary, but the predictability and connection they provide are important for good sleep, having repeatedly been shown to help sleep at every age, from infancy to adult. What does a good bedtime routine look like at this age? Here is an example:

> 6.30 p.m. – thirty minutes' playtime together
> 7 p.m. – offer a small bedtime snack
> 7.15 p.m. – bath time and teeth brushing
> 7.30 p.m. – change into pyjamas and prepare bedroom
>   for sleep
> 7.40 p.m. – bedtime story
> 7.45 p.m. – cuddles and goodnight kisses
> 8 p.m. – sleep onset

Ensure correct nutrient consumption   If your four-year-old is picky or follows a special diet (vegetarian or vegan, for example), it is important to make sure that they get enough iron, omega-3 and magnesium in their diet. A deficiency in any of these can have a negative impact on sleep: iron can cause restlessness during sleep, and you may notice your child thrashing around a lot in bed; omega-3 is related to parasomnias (such as night terrors); and magnesium impacts on the ability to relax.

Use sleep-friendly lighting   As discussed earlier (see page 124), lighting in the two hours before bedtime and overnight can impact children's sleep. Be careful about exposure to screens (ideally, there should be no screen time after 6 p.m.) and consider the lighting used around your home. Use dim lighting only in the run-up to bedtime (including in the bathroom) and only red lighting in your child's bedroom, especially if they prefer to have a night light.

Set clear boundaries Toddlerhood isn't the only age when children test boundaries – this continues throughout childhood. Setting clear boundaries around bedtime – what is expected and when – helps children to feel safe and secure and keeps their daily routine predictable. Relaxing boundaries too much around bedtime (giving in to requests or being too flexible) can cause difficulties with sleep. Sticking calmly and respectfully to bedtime boundaries is the best solution.

Use comfort cues Helping children to feel safe and secure through comfort cues will not only help them to fall asleep more easily, but also reassure them more when they wake in the night. Here, think about soothing music for them to fall asleep to, cuddling up with a favourite teddy bear and snuggling a soft blanket together while they fall asleep, so they associate the blanket with you.

Moving to independent bedtimes

This is a common age for parents and carers to want to move towards more independent bedtimes, perhaps simply giving their child a kiss and leaving them to go to sleep alone. While

> The only thing worth stealing is a kiss from
> a sleeping child.
> J. H. Oldham, Scottish missionary

this goal is understandable, after four years of parentcentric bedtimes, it is sadly not developmentally appropriate. At four years old, children cannot regulate their emotions well and self-settle or self-soothe. Bedtime, or rather being left alone in the relative dark, is a vulnerable time for children from an evolutionary perspective. It is in a young child's nature to cling to their parent or carer – the person who will keep them safe in the dark. Independent bedtimes will happen naturally as children grow, but there are a few steps you can take to work towards them at this age:

A bedtime friend to care for Have you ever noticed that if you're scared of something but caring for another, such as your child, your fear lessens? You can use this principle to help children at bedtime by giving them a special 'bedtime friend' (a teddy bear or similar) to care for, so that their anxiety and fear are transferred on to the toy. Remind them that if the bear gets scared, it is their job to look after them, saying something like, 'If he wakes and he's scared or lonely, can you give him a big squeeze and tell him that it's OK to go back to sleep?' The hope here is that they will comfort the bear if they themselves are feeling anxious or lonely.

Popping in and out One of the keys to surviving separation anxiety, for both parents and children, is to separate in small, well-timed doses. Using this concept at bedtime can be really helpful. Once your child is tucked up and their bedtime routine is complete, say something like, 'Oh, I need to go to the toilet. I'll be back in a minute.' Then leave the room and stay out for as long as they don't cry or call for you. If they do cry or call out, go straight back to their room and say, 'It's OK, I'm here, don't worry, I'm always here if you need me.' Once they are calm say, 'Oh no, I didn't turn off the tap, back in a minute' and repeat. Initially, your 'pop outs' may only be a minute or two long. Your aim is not for the child to go to sleep while you are out of the room, but just to be comfortable in your absence. Ultimately, they may fall asleep while you are out, but don't expect that to happen for at least the first few weeks.

Guided relaxation Child-friendly guided relaxation recordings can be a great tool to help with independent sleep onset. They work to take the child's mind off 'going to sleep' and help them to relax and feel calm in your absence. When choosing a recording, aim for one that isn't exhilarating in any way (no flying or chasing things) and, ideally, one that teaches them new coping strategies for sleep, so that the effect builds the more times that they listen to it (see Resources, page 257). Start the recording once you have tucked your child in and said goodnight. For the first week or so, lie with them until they are asleep, then you can try to leave just before you put the recording on, or part way into it.

Hopefully, with these three tips (and a lot of patience) you can look forward to kissing your child goodnight and leaving them to drift off to sleep independently – but most importantly, happily – in the not-too-distant future and for many years to come.

Parent Observation 'My daughter needed me to hug her to sleep until she was about five or six years old. I can't lie and say I didn't find it irritating at times, but there was something lovely about seeing her drift off to sleep in my arms. Now she's seven, I really miss the bedtime cuddles; she just gives me a kiss and waves me off!'

Social and psychological development from four to five years

Your four-year-old is a highly sociable little being. Between the ages of four and five they move into the stage of co-operative play, when children are actively interested in the play activities of others, as well as in the other children themselves. The emergence of co-operative play indicates the child has achieved a level of social maturity that includes a more developed theory of mind (see page 214).

Children at this stage understand much more about social interactions and have emerging empathy for their peers. Their

PARENTING Q&A

Q. *My son behaves so well at school all day and his teacher says he is a little angel, but when we get home his behaviour is terrible. He shouts and kicks me. What am I doing wrong?*

A. *Your son is experiencing something known as after-school restraint collapse. This means that he is doing well to keep a lid on his big emotions all day while he is at school, behaving as the school expects. But when he gets home, he knows it is safe to lift that lid and release the pent-up emotions, because he knows that you love and support him regardless of how he behaves. It can be difficult to cope with, but rather than being an indication of something you have done wrong, after-school restraint collapse is testament to your nurturing parenting and how secure your son feels with you.*

Why rewards are ineffective as discipline

The use of rewards, such as sticker charts, as a discipline tool for children stems from techniques of behaviour modification that have been popular for almost a century – the same model that gave us the basis for modern-day dog training. But while rewards may help to train our dogs, these methods are ineffective when it comes to disciplining children. Rewards don't deal with the cause of the issue or resolve the difficult feelings underlying the behaviour. They just palliate them, usually producing quick, but temporary results, which can (and does) mean far worse behaviour in the future.

The biggest misconception about behaviour when using rewards is that the child can control and change it – the assumption being that the problem is not one of ability, but motivation. But we know that young children have an immature prefrontal cortex and, as such, they cannot control their behaviour in the way that adults can. Therefore, a discipline method that focuses solely on motivation, disregarding ability, is always going to be ineffective.

Rewards work on extrinsic (external) motivation. They work quickly (i.e. the temporary positive result gained through short-term compliance), but any positive effects are very superficial. For a real change to take place, parents and carers need to work with a child's intrinsic (internal) motivation, and, unfortunately, rewarding damages this. Basically, the more we reward a child for doing something, the less likely they are to do it in the future (unless we keep rewarding them – and increasing the reward value). The child is not learning 'right from wrong' or becoming a better person this way; instead, they comply while the reward is on offer – but when you remove it (or offer one

> that doesn't tempt them enough) you lose their compli-
> ance.
>   The solution here is focusing on understanding your
> child's neurological abilities, investigating the cause of their
> difficult behaviour, teaching and guiding them to better
> behaviour and being a great role model to encourage
> intrinsic motivation.

social skills are still immature compared to an adult's, though, and combined with their incomplete brain development, this means it is likely that lots of bickering between friends will occur. Four-year-olds also aren't naturally good at sharing or turn taking. These aren't flaws – again, they are stages of development. The best way to help them learn to make and keep friendships and to tackle issues that come up is to role model empathy and compassion and teach them how to take turns at home. Punishing a child for not willingly sharing is ineffective – it just punishes them for having a child's brain.

Separation anxiety starts to lessen at this age, as children begin to recognise the idea of time. This means that your four-year-old comprehends that when you leave them you will return at a later time, and although they may not appreciate the intricacies of minutes and hours, they do understand explanations such as 'I'll see you after lunch'.

Magical thinking – why children struggle with logic

At this age, your four-year-old will likely believe that they can influence situations because of their thoughts. For instance, if they really want to receive a gift and somebody buys it for them

Never ever doubt in magic. The purest honest thoughts
come from children, ask any child if they believe in magic
and they will tell you the truth.
Scott Dixon, author

(with no knowledge that the child wanted it), they will believe
that their wishes and thoughts made the gift materialise. This
type of thought pattern is known as 'magical thinking' and
lasts until children are around ten years old. Magical thinking isn't just confined to a child's thoughts, though – they
may also believe that performing a certain action or saying a
certain word can make something happen. Magical thinking
helps to explain why young children are drawn to magic and
magical beings, such as fairies, unicorns and wizards.

The downside of this thought process is that children
can blame themselves if something bad happens. If they

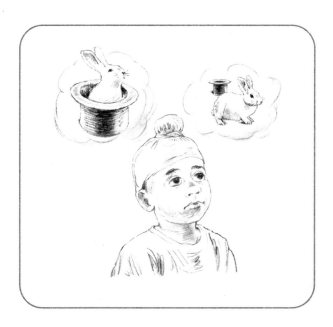

accidentally break something, for example, and then you become sick the next day, they may believe that their behaviour made this happen. By understanding magical thinking and children's lack of adult-style logic, parents and carers can help to reassure them in times of anxiety and sadness.

Language and communication from four to five years

Your four-year-old's speech will be coming on in leaps and bounds. They will be speaking in more complex sentences containing several words, including connecting ones, such as 'when' and 'and'. Their speech will also improve grammatically at this age, with their sentence structure maturing.

Your four-year-old will become more adept at telling you about their feelings and needs, saying, 'I'm hungry', 'I'm scared' and 'I'm tired', for example, and they will increasingly use adjectives to explain things in more detail.

Children's vocabulary at this stage will likely include words that refer to the past and future – for instance, they may say, 'I remember when we saw the horses' or, 'When we go on holiday next week'. This new skill indicates a change in their memory and understanding of time, as they are able to recognise and verbalise the differences between past, present and future.

Although your child's vocabulary is expanding rapidly, they still understand far more words than they can say at this age.

The focus now is on helping children to develop their storytelling abilities (that is explaining events, not reading from a book) and to understand turn taking in conversations and social rules surrounding language (speaking at an appro-

PARENTING Q&A

Q. *What should we do when our son mispronounces words? Some of his mispronunciations are so sweet I don't want to correct him.*

A. *Mispronunciation of words is very common at this age. Instead of correcting, just gently repeat the word back as it should be said. So if your son says 'bisgetti' instead of 'spaghetti', for example, you could say, 'Yes, you like the spaghetti, don't you?'*

priate volume or waiting until an existing conversation is finished before speaking, for example). Holding regular conversations with them, asking them to explain what they can see when you are out and about, pointing out pictures in a book or summarising a TV programme are all good ways to improve their storytelling. This will also advance their conversation skills, as they learn the rhythm of turn taking. Social rules take a bit longer to acquire, largely as they are the result of emotion regulation and impulse control, but games where you teach them the difference in speaking volumes (with shouting, talking loudly, indoor quiet voices and whispering, in the style of 'Simon Says') are a fun way to encourage a quieter voice when necessary.

FUN FACT

By the time children are five years old, their vocabulary can reach 10,000 words, as compared with the average adult's, which is 20,000 to 35,000 words.

> **Parent Observation** My son used to speak really loudly. In fact, sometimes he was so loud it was like he was shouting all the time. For a while, we thought he was just loud, but then a friend suggested we got his hearing checked. The doctor diagnosed him with glue ear, where his ear canals were bunged up with fluid. We were referred to the hospital who fitted him with grommets to help the fluid drain and he was instantly so much quieter once he could hear properly.'

If you have concerns about your child's speech, then do speak to their preschool or school for advice. You could also ask your GP or health visitor for a referral to a speech and language therapist. It is always better to seek help as early as possible because early intervention leads to the most successful results. Speech therapy for young children is a fun activity, directed around play, and most children enjoy their sessions.

Play ideas for four to five years

Your four-year-old will spend more time sitting when they start school, so it is important to encourage as much free movement and activity as possible when they are at home. Spending time playing in nature, whatever the weather, encouraging running, jumping, climbing, dancing and riding a bike are important for your four-year-old.

This is a good time for your child to start to learn a musical instrument, with good choices including the recorder, piano and guitar. This isn't so much about creating a future musical genius, but rather, a love of music, so hold back on strict formal lessons and encourage fun and exploration instead.

> There is no such thing as bad weather, only
> inappropriate clothing.
> *Sir Ranulph Fiennes, British explorer*

Imaginative play comes into its own during this period, fully embracing a child's magical thinking. Creating a dressing-up box (using your old clothing, jewellery, accessories and shoes) is time well invested. Children of this age get as much fun out of selecting their own costumes from discarded adult clothing as they do from expensive shop-bought dressing up costumes. In fact, there is better play value in homemade costumes that can be used for a variety of different characters than a commercial one intended for just one.

Finally, this is a good age to introduce turn-taking games. Although children are likely to struggle with this (and tantrums will often ensue), teaching them to share time through play is a lovely, organic way to encourage their social skills. Just remember to keep your expectations of their abilities and behaviour age appropriate. When they do inevitably tantrum and struggle with taking turns, they are not doing so because they are selfish or being naughty, they are struggling because of immature brain development.

FUN FACT

Children who learn to play an instrument in early childhood show better literacy and language skills as they get older; they also tend to have better self-esteem than those who do not.

The theory of loose parts

Loose parts, or multiple small objects that can be used in play, help to encourage open-ended learning, whereby children learn to use the same items in myriad different ways. This helps them to develop problem-solving skills, encourages their imaginations and keeps them entertained for longer.

Here are some suggestions for loose parts that can be used in play:

Blocks of wood	Empty yoghurt pots
Rocks and pebbles	Feathers
Wooden lollipop sticks	Straws
Leaves and flowers	Pipe cleaners
Pieces of fabric	Buttons
Toy animals or cars	Plastic gutter tubing
Stacking cups or containers	Funnels and pouring
Shells	jugs
Pine cones	Sand or mud
Empty kitchen or toilet-roll	Rice or dried pasta
tubes	Water

Children are left to arrange the loose parts into any play scenario that inspires them. Some may create specific scenes, while others may just enjoy building and connecting the items in a way that is meaningful to them. Loose-parts play is almost always more entertaining to children than specific toys or organised activities.

Play is the highest expression of human development
in childhood, for it alone is the free expression of
what is in a child's soul.
Friedrich Froebel, German educator

Recommended toys

Toy selections at this age reflect maturing fine motor skills, magical thinking and increasing social skills. Here are some good choices:

- **Remote-controlled toys** – children of this age love to play with remote-controlled cars, helicopters and robots, which boost levels of autonomy and help fine motor skill development

- **A children's cookery set** – with a child-sized apron and child-safe knife, so they can help you in the kitchen

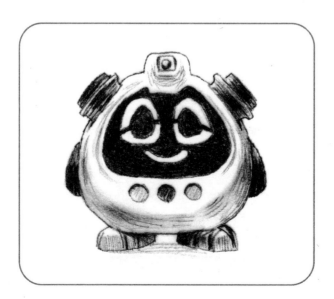

- **A den-building kit** – to use in a local nature spot to encourage a love of the outdoors

- **Dressing-up outfits** – to inspire their imagination and feed into their innate magical thinking

- **Co-operative board games** – to encourage turn taking, but also working together to achieve a goal (given that co-operative board games are ones where the whole team wins, rather than one player)

- **Jigsaw puzzles** – children can handle jigsaw puzzles with around thirty-five to fifty pieces at this age

- **A crate containing a selection of interesting 'loose parts'** – for children to create their own play

Even though your child is getting older and more independent, their favourite plaything is still you. Perhaps the most fun, enjoyable and, indeed, beneficial way to entertain them is by playing with them. Roughhousing, often called 'horse play', is incredibly popular with children of this age. Intense, physical play with adults and carers helps a child to deepen connection, fulfils their need for attention, improves their gross motor

> When we roughhouse with our kids, we model for them how someone bigger and stronger holds back. We teach them self-control, fairness and empathy. We let them win, which gives them confidence and demonstrates that winning isn't everything. We show them how much can be accomplished by co-operation and how to constructively channel competitive energy so that it doesn't take over.
> *Laurence Cohen, author of* Playful Parenting

skills and improves their self-esteem. Research has even shown that children who regularly roughhouse with their parents or carers are less aggressive, have better friendships at school and do better academically than those children who do not.[6]

It is fitting that we end this chapter with the emphasis on you, the parent or carer, because it is you who gives your child roots and strong foundations – the underpinnings that, ultimately, lead to their flourishing wings of confidence and independence. Your four-year-old is very much a social butterfly today because of the solid base they have built with you – not just through play, but through the everyday interactions that we, as adults, may consider monotonous or mundane, but to our children are anything but.

> Behind every young child who believes in himself
> is a parent who believed first.
> *Matthew Jacobson, historian*

A Closing Note

The beginning of a new life is possibly the most wondrous thing we could ever be blessed to observe. To be *in* a child's life as they grow, both physically and emotionally, and to have a direct impact on that growth is mind-blowing. There are so many 'firsts', so much wonder and so much excitement and pride. These months and years can also bring with them feelings of self-doubt, however, as we realise that this little person's life – their physical and emotional development – depends upon us and our actions. I hope this book has helped you to realise that children don't need a mountain of special toys or expensive classes to flourish, though; what they need is far simpler than that – it's you.

Never underestimate how powerful and influential you are for your child. Your love, support and nurturance – during the everyday otherwise mundane moments – are what helps them to grow and develop. Sometimes, as parents and carers of young children, we berate ourselves for not doing enough, for not being enough. But to our babies and children we are more than enough; we are their whole world.

I hope that this book has helped you to see how important and amazing you are, as well as giving you an insight into the wondrous developments that your child has already made and will continue to make with your help.

Sarah

Resources

Other books by Sarah Ockwell-Smith

On behaviour and discipline:
The Gentle Discipline Book

On weaning and eating:
The Gentle Eating Book

On improving baby and child sleep:
The Gentle Sleep Book

On preparing to start school:
The Starting School Book

On potty training:
The Gentle Potty Training Book

On parental emotions and handling stress and triggers:
How to be a Calm Parent

Music and Relaxation Recordings for Baby and Child Sleep

'Gentle Sleep Music for Babies' by Ian Ockwell-Smith,
    available on Amazon, Apple Music, iTunes and Spotify

'Gentle Sleep Relaxation for Children' by Sarah
    Ockwell-Smith, available on Amazon, Apple Music,
    iTunes and Spotify

Sarah's Social Media

Website and newsletter: www.sarahockwell-smith.com

Facebook: www.facebook.com/sarahockwellsmithauthor

Instagram: www.instagram.com/sarahockwellsmith

Twitter: www.twitter.com/thebabyexpert

YouTube videos: www.youtube.com/c/sarahockwellsmith

Support Organisations and Professionals

Autism support: the National Autistic Society
www.autism.org.uk

ADHD support: the ADHD Foundation
www.adhdfoundation.org.uk

Breastfeeding support: LaLeche League
www.laleche.org.uk

the Breastfeeding Network
www.breastfeedingnetwork.org.uk

Dyslexia support: British Dyslexia Association
www.bdadyslexia.org.uk

Dyspraxia support: Dyspraxia Foundation
www.dyspraxiafoundation.org.uk

Prematurity support: Bliss
www.bliss.org.uk

Language-development support: ICAN
www.ican.org.uk

Tongue-tie support: find a practitioner at:
www.tongue-tie.co.uk

References

Chapter 1

1 Konkel, L. (2018), 'The brain before birth: using fMRI to explore the secrets of fetal neurodevelopment, *Environmental Health Perspectives*, 126(11).

2 Ackerman, S. (1992), 'The development and shaping of the brain', Washington (DC), National Academies Press (US).

3 Salomon, L. J., Bernard, J. P. and Ville, Y. (2007), 'Estimation of fetal weight: reference range at 20–36 weeks' gestation and comparison with actual birth-weight reference range', *Ultrasound Obstetrics and Gynecology*, 29, pp. 550–55.

4 Condon, J. C., Jeyasuria, P., Faust, J. M. and Mendelson, C. R. (2004), 'Surfactant protein secreted by the maturing mouse fetal lung acts as a hormone that signals the initiation of parturition', *Proceedings of the National Academy of Sciences of the United States of America*, 101(14), pp. 4978–83.

5 Polettini. J., Behnia, F., Taylor, B. D., Saade, G. R., Taylor, R. N., et al. (2015), 'Telomere fragment induced amnion cell senescence: a contributor to parturition?', *PLOS One*, 10(9), e0137188.

6 Spahn, J., Callahan, E., Spill, M., et al. (2019), 'Influence of maternal diet on flavor transfer to amniotic fluid and breast milk and children's responses: a systematic review', *American Journal of Clinical Nutrition*, 109 (supplement 1), pp. 1003S–26S.

7 Johnson, S., Pastuschek, J., Rödel, J., et al. (2018), 'The placenta – worth trying? Human maternal placentophagia: possible benefit and potential risks', *Geburtshilfe Frauenheilkd*, 78(9), pp. 846–52.

8 Suwanrath, C. and Suntharasaj, T. (2010), 'Sleep-wake cycles in

   normal fetuses', *Archives of Gynecology and Obstetrics*, 281(3),
   pp. 449–54.

9 Schwab, K., Groh, T., Schwab, M., et al. (2009), 'Nonlinear analysis
   and modeling of cortical activation and deactivation patterns in the
   immature fetal electrocorticogram', *Chaos*, 19(1), 015111.

10 DiPietro, J., Kivlighan, K., Costigan, K., et al. (2010), 'Prenatal
   antecedents of newborn neurological maturation', *Child
   Development*, 81(1), pp. 115–30.

11 Werner, E. A., Myers, M. M., Fifer, W. P., Cheng, B., Fang, Y., Allen, R.
   and Monk, C. (2007), 'Prenatal predictors of infant temperament',
   Developmental Psychobiology, 49, pp. 474–84.

12 Poćwierz-Marciniak, I. and Harciarek, M. (2021), 'The Effect of
   musical stimulation and mother's voice on the early development
   of musical abilities: a neuropsychological perspective', *International
   Journal of Environmental Research and Public Health*, 18, p. 8467.

13 Institute Marques (2018), 'Which music stimulates your baby?',
   Barcelona, Spain.

14 Mampe, B., Friederici, A., Wermke, K., et al. (2009), 'Newborns' cry
   melody is shaped by their native language', *Current Biology*, 19(23),
   pp. 1994–7.

15 Lee G. Y. and Kisilevsky, B. S. (2014), 'Fetuses respond to father's
   voice but prefer mother's voice after birth', *Developmental
   Psychobiology*, Jan, 56(1), pp. 1–11.

Chapter 2

1 Wellmann, S. and Buhrer, C. (2012), 'Who plays the strings in
   newborn analgesia at birth, vasopressin or oxytocin?' *Frontiers in
   Neuroscience*, 6.

2 Power, C., Williams, C. and Brown, A. (2019), 'Does childbirth
   experience affect infant behaviour? Exploring the perceptions of
   maternity care providers', *Midwifery*, 78, pp. 131–9.

3 Moore, Elizabeth R., et al. (2012), 'Early skin-to-skin contact for
   mothers and their healthy newborn infants', *Cochrane Database of
   Systematic Reviews*, 5(5).

4 Lundstrom, J., Mathe, A., Schaal, B., et al. (2013), 'Maternal status

regulates cortical responses to the body odor of newborns', *Frontiers in Psychology*, 4, p. 597.

5 Varendi, Heili (2001), 'Breast odour as the only maternal stimulus elicits crawling towards the odour source', *Acta Paediatrica*, 90, pp. 372–5.

6 Macfarlane, A. (1975), 'Olfaction in the development of social preferences in the human neonate', *Ciba Foundation Symposium*, (33), pp. 103–17.

7 Zanardo, V. and Straface, G. (2015), 'The higher temperature in the areola supports the natural progression of the birth to breastfeeding continuum', *PLOS One*, 10(3).

8 Holland, D., Chang, L., Ernst, T. M., et al. (2014), 'Structural growth trajectories and rates of change in the first 3 months of infant brain development', *JAMA Neurology*, 71(10), pp. 1266–74.

9 Ibid.

10 Lohmann, C. and Bonhoeffer, T. (2008), 'A role for local calcium signaling in rapid synaptic partner selection by dendritic filopodia', *Neuron*, 59, pp. 253–60.

11 Maitre, N., Key, A. and Chorna, O. (2017), 'The dual nature of early life experience on somatosensory processing in the human infant brain', *Current Biology*, 27(7), e1048–54.

12 Dehaene-Lambertz, G., Montavont, A., Jobert, A., Allirol, L., et al. (2010), 'Language or music, mother or Mozart? Structural and environmental influences on infants' language networks', *Brain and Language*, 114(2), pp. 53–65.

13 Barrera, M. and Maurer, D. (1981), 'Recognition of mother's photographed face by the three-month old infant', *Society for Research in Child Development,* 52(2), pp. 714–16.

14 Sokoloff, G., Dooley, J., Glanz, R., et al. (2021), 'Twitches emerge postnatally during quiet sleep in human infants and are synchronized with sleep spindles', *Current Biology*, 31(15): e3426–32.

15 Shimizu. M., Park, H., and Greenfield, P. M. (2014), 'Infant sleeping arrangements and cultural values among contemporary Japanese mothers', *Frontiers in Psychology*, 5, p. 718.

16 Ellwood, J., Draper-Rodi, J. and Carnes, D. (2020), 'Comparison

of common interventions for the treatment of infantile colic: a systematic review of reviews and guidelines', *BMJ Open,* 10: e035405.

17 Shimizu. M., Park, H., and Greenfield, P. M. (2014), 'Infant sleeping arrangements and cultural values among contemporary Japanese mothers', *Frontiers in Psychology*, 5, p. 718.

18 Luby, J. (2015), 'The importance of early nurturance for social development', *Journal of the American Academy of Child and Adolescent Psychiatry*, 54(12), pp. 972–3.

19 Feldman, R., Bamberger, E. and Kanat-Maymon, Y. (2013), 'Parent-specific reciprocity from infancy to adolescence shapes children's social competence and dialogical skills', *Attachment and Human Development*, 13, 15(4), pp. 407–23.

20 Underdown, A., Barlow, J., Chung, V. and Stewart-Brown, S. (2006), 'Massage intervention for promoting mental and physical health in infants aged under six months', *Cochrane Database Systematic Review*, 18(4).

21 Gunnar, M. R. (2006), 'Social regulation of stress in early childhood'. In McCartney, K. and Phillips, D. (eds), *Blackwell Handbook of Early Childhood Development*, Malden: Blackwell Publishing (pp. 106–25).

Chapter 3

1 Addabbo, M. and Turati C. (2020), 'Binding actions and emotions in the infant's brain', *Society for Neuroscience*, 15(4), pp. 470–76.

2 Parise, E., Friederici, A. D. and Striano, T. (2010), 'Did you call me? 5-month-old infants own name guides their attention', *PLOS One*, 3, 5(12).

3 Kringelbach, M., Stark, E., Alexander, C., et al. (2016), 'On cuteness: unlocking the parental brain and beyond', *Trends in Cognitive Sciences*, 20(7), pp. 545–8.

4 Yang, J., Kanazawa, S., Yamaguchi, M. K. and Motoyoshi, I. (2015), 'Pre-constancy vision in infants', *Current Biology*, 25(24), pp. 3209–12.

5 Romandini, M., Oxilia, G. and Bortolini, E. (2020), 'A late Neanderthal tooth from northeastern Italy', *Journal of Human Evolution*, 147, Oct., 102867.

6   Macknin, M. L., Piedmonte, M., Jacobs, J. and Skibinski, C. (2000), 'Symptoms associated with infant teething: a prospective study', *Pediatrics*, 105(4 pt 1), pp. 747–52.

7   Liem, D. G. (2017), 'Infants' and children's salt taste perception and liking: a review', *Nutrients*, 9(9), 1011.

8   Henderson, J. (2010), 'Sleeping through the night: the consolidation of self-regulated sleep across the first year of life', *Pediatrics*, 126(5), pp. 1081–7.

9   Iglowstein, I., Jenni, O., Molinari, L., et al. (2003), 'Sleep duration from infancy to adolescence: reference values and generational trends', *Pediatrics*, 111(2), pp. 302–7.

10 Pennestri, M., Burdayron, R., Kenny, S., et al. (2020), 'Sleeping through the night or through the nights?' *Sleep Medicine*, 76, p. 98.

11 Brown, A. and Harries, V. (2015), 'Infant sleep and night feeding patterns during later infancy: association with breastfeeding frequency, daytime complementary food intake, and infant weight', *Breastfeeding Medicine*, 10(5), pp. 246–52.

12 Feldman, R., Bamberger, E. and Kanat-Maymon, Y. (2013), 'Parent specific reciprocity from infancy to adolescence shapes children's social competence and dialogical skills', *Attachment and Human Development*, 15, pp. 407–23.

13 Hoicka, E., Soy Telli, B., Prouten, E., et al. (2021), 'The early humor survey (EHS): a reliable parent-report measure of humor development for 1- to 47-month-olds', *Behavior Research Methods*.

Chapter 4

1   Tierney, A. and Nelson, C. (2009), 'Brain development and the role of experience in the early years', *Zero to Three*, 30(2), pp. 9–13.

2   Imada, T., Zhang, Y., Cheour, M., et al. (2006), 'Infant speech perception activates Broca's area: a developmental magnetoencephalography study', *Neuroreport*, 17(10), pp. 957–62.

3   Grossman, T., Obereker, R., Koch, S., et al. (2010), 'The developmental origins of voice processing in the human brain', 65(6), pp. 852–8.

4   Meltzoff, A., Ramirez, R., Saby, J., et al. (2018), 'Infant brain

responses to felt and observed touch of hands and feet: an MEG study', *Developmental Science*, 21(5), e12651.

5 Sen, M. G., Yonas, A. and Knill, D. C. (2001), 'Development of infants' sensitivity to surface contour information for spatial layout', *Perception*, 30(2), pp. 167–76.

6 Gibson, E. J. and Walk, R. D. (1960), 'The "visual cliff"', *Scientific American*, 202(4), pp. 64–71.

7 Zentner, M. and Eerola, T. (2010), 'Rhythmic engagement with music in infancy', *Proceedings of the National Academy of Sciences*, 107(13), pp. 5768–73.

8 Paavonen, J., Saarenpää-Heikkilä, O., Morales-Munoz, I., et al. (2020), 'Normal sleep development in infants: findings from two large birth cohorts', *Sleep Medicine*, 69, pp. 145–54.

9 Pennestri, M., Burdayron, R., Kenny, S., et al. (2020), 'Sleeping through the night or through the nights?' *Sleep Medicine*, 76, pp. 98–103.

10 Price, A. M., Wake, M., Ukoumunne, O. C. and Hiscock, H. (2012), 'Five-year follow-up of harms and benefits of behavioral infant sleep intervention: randomized trial', *Pediatrics*, 130(4), pp. 643–51.

11 Filippi, C., Cannon, E., Fox, N., et al. (2016), 'Motor system activation predicts goal imitation in 7-month-old infants', *Psychological Science*, 27(5), pp. 675–84.

12 Wynn, K. and Bloom, P. (2014), 'The moral baby', in Killen, M. and Smetana, J. G. (eds), *Handbook of Moral Development*, Psychology Press, pp. 435–53.

Chapter 5

1 A. Bernier, F. Dégeilh, É. Leblanc, et al. (2019), 'Mother–infant interaction and child brain morphology: a multidimensional approach to maternal sensitivity in Infancy', *Developmental Cognitive Neuroscience*, 24(2), pp. 120–38.

2 Vöhringer, I., Kolling, T. and Graf, F. (2017), 'The development of implicit memory from infancy to childhood: on average performance levels and interindividual differences', *Child Development*, 89(2), pp. 370–82.

3 Peterson, C. (2021), 'What is your earliest memory? It depends', *Memory*, 29(6), pp. 811–22.

4 MacNeill, L. A., Ram, N., Bell, M. A., Fox, N. A. and Pérez-Edgar, K. (2018), 'Trajectories of infants' biobehavioral development: timing and rate of a-not-b performance gains and EEG maturation', *Child Development*, 89(3), pp. 711–24.

5 Sullivan, S. and Birch, L. (1994), 'Infant dietary experience and acceptance of solid foods', *Pediatrics*, 93(2), pp. 271–7.

6 Armstrong, K. L., Quinn, R. A. and Dadds, M. R. (1994), 'The sleep patterns of normal children', *Medical Journal of Australia,* 161(3), pp. 202–6.

7 Mindell, J., Leichman, E., Composto, J., et al. (2016), 'Development of infant and toddler sleep patterns: real-world data from a mobile application', *Journal of Sleep Research*, 25(5), pp. 508–16.

8 Brown, A. and Harries, V. (2015), 'Infant sleep and night feeding patterns during later infancy: association with breastfeeding frequency, daytime complementary food intake, and infant weight', *Breastfeeding Medicine*, 10(5), pp. 246–52.

9 Wright, H. and Lack, L. (2001), 'Effect of light wavelength on suppression and phase delay of the melatonin rhythm', *Chronobiology International*,18(5), pp. 801–8

10 Mountain, G., Cahill, J. and Thorpe, H. (2017), 'Sensitivity and attachment interventions in early childhood: a systematic review and meta-analysis', *Infant Behaviour and Development*, 46, pp. 14–32.

11 Bowlby, J. (1969), *Attachment and Loss* (OKS Print), New York: Basic Books.

12 Syrnyk, C.and Meints, K. (2017), 'Bye-bye mummy – word comprehension in 9-month-old infants', *British Journal of Developmental Psychology*, 35(2), pp. 202–17.

13 Tardif, T., Fletcher, P. and Kaciroti, N. (2008), 'Baby's first 10 words', *Developmental Psychology*, 44(4), pp. 929–38.

14 Kuhl, P. K. (2004), 'Early language acquisition: Cracking the speech code', *Nature Reviews Neuroscience*, 5, pp. 831–43.

15 Piazza, E., Hasenfratz, L., Hasson, U., et al, (2019), 'Infant and adult

brains are coupled to the dynamics of natural communication',
Psychological Science, 31(1), pp. 6–17.

Chapter 6

1 Shonkoff, J. P. and Phillips, D. A. (eds) (2000), 'From neurons to
   neighborhoods: the science of early childhood development',
   National Academies Press.

2 Ibid.

3 Zhao, C. and Kuhl, P. (2016), 'Musical intervention enhances
   infants' neural processing of temporal structure in music and
   speech', *Proceedings of the National Academy of Sciences,* 113(19),
   pp. 5212–17.

4 Jones, E., Goodwin, A., Orekhova, A., et al. (2020), 'Infant EEG theta
   modulation predicts childhood intelligence', *Scientific Reports,* 10,
   article: 11232.

5 Jarvis, I., Davis, Z., Sbihi, H., et al. (2021), 'Assessing the association
   between lifetime exposure to greenspace and early childhood
   development and the mediation effects of air pollution and noise
   in Canada: a population-based birth cohort study', *Lancet Planetary
   Health,* 5(10).

6 Avila, W., Pordeus, I., Paiva, S., et al. (2015), 'Breast and bottle
   feeding as risk factors for dental caries: a systematic review and
   meta-analysis', *PLOS One,* 18, 10(11).

7 No authors listed (2016), 'Breastfeeding: achieving the new normal',
   Lancet, 387 (10017).

8 Lawrence, R. M. and Lawrence, R. A. (2011) 'Breastfeeding: more
   than just good nutrition', *Pediatric Review,* 32(7), pp. 267–80.

9 Ibid.

10 Onyango, A. W., Receveur, O. and Esrey, S. A. (2002), 'The
    contribution of breast milk to toddler diets in western Kenya',
    Bulletin of the World Health Organization, 80(4), pp. 292–9.

11 Duazo, P., Avila, J. and Kuzawa, C. (2010), 'Breastfeeding and later
    psychosocial development in the Philippines', *Human Biology,* 22(6),
    pp. 725–30.

12 Scher, A. (1991), 'A longitudinal study of night waking in the first year', *Child Care Health and Development*, 17(5), pp. 295–302.

13 Armstrong, K. L., Quinn, R. A. and Dadds, M. R. (1994), 'The sleep patterns of normal children', *Medical Journal of Australia*, 161(3), pp. 202–6.

14 Mindell, J., Leichman, E., Composto, J., et al. (2016), 'Development of infant and toddler sleep patterns: real-world data from a mobile application', *Journal of Sleep Research*, 25(5), pp. 508–16.

15 Ainsworth, M. D. S. and Bell, S. M. (1970), 'Attachment, exploration and separation: illustrated by the behavior of one-year-olds in a strange situation', *Child Development,* 41, pp. 49–67.

16 Main, M. and Solomon, J. (1990), 'Procedures for identifying infants as disorganized/disoriented during the Ainsworth Strange Situation'. In Greenberg, M. T., Cicchetti, D. and Cummings, E. M. (eds), *Attachment in the Preschool Years*, University of Chicago Press, pp. 121–60.

17 Broder, E. (2008), 'Attachment from infancy to adulthood: the major longitudinal studies', *Journal of the Canadian Academy of Child and Adolescent Psychiatry*, 17(3), p. 161.

Chapter 7

1 Dekaban, A. and Sadowsky, D. (1978), 'Changes in brain weights during the span of human life: relation of brain weights to body heights and body weights', *Annals of Neurology*, 4, pp. 345–56.

2 Perry, L., Samuelson, L. and Burdinie, J. (2013), 'Highchair philosophers: the impact of seating context-dependent exploration on children's naming biases', *Developmental Science*, 17(5), pp. 757–65.

3 Cardona Cano, S., Tiemeier, H. and Van Hoken, D. (2015), 'Trajectories of picky eating during childhood: a general population study', *International Journal of Eating Disorders*, 48(6), pp. 570–9.

4 Williams, S. and Horst, J. (2014), 'Goodnight book: sleep consolidation improves word learning via storybooks', *Frontiers in Psychology*, Mar. 4(5), p. 184.

5 Iglowstein, I., Molinari, L. and Largo, R. (2003), 'Sleep duration from infancy to adolescence: reference values and generational trends', *Pediatrics*, 111(2), pp. 302–7.

6 Ibid.

7 Horváth, K., and Plunkett, K. (2018), 'Spotlight on daytime napping during early childhood', *Nature and Science of Sleep*, 10, pp. 97–104; Acebo, C., Sadeh, A., Seifer, R., et al. (2005), 'Sleep/wake patterns derived from activity monitoring and maternal report for healthy 1- to 5-year-old children', *Sleep*, 28(12), pp. 1568–77.

8 Mindell, J., Leichman, E., Composto, J., et al. (2016), 'Development of infant and toddler sleep patterns: real-world data from a mobile application', *Journal of Sleep Research*, 25(5), pp. 508–16.

9 Paavonen, E., Saarenpää-Heikkilä, O., Morales-Munoz, I., et al. (2020), 'Normal sleep development in infants: findings from two large birth cohorts', *Sleep Medicine*, 69, pp. 145–54.

10 Sisterhen, L. and Wy, P. (2021), *Temper Tantrums*, StatPearls Publishing, Florida, USA.

Chapter 8

1 Bunge, S. and Zelazo, P. (2006), 'A brain-based account of the development of rule use in childhood', *Current Directions in Psychological Science*, 15(3), pp. 118–21.

2 Sakai, J. (2020), 'Core concept: how synaptic pruning shapes neural wiring during development and, possibly, in disease', *Proceedings of the National Academy of Sciences*, 117(28), pp. 16096–9.

3 Molfese, V. J., Rudasill, K. M., Prokasky, A., et al. (2015), 'Relations between toddler sleep characteristics, sleep problems, and temperament', *Developmental Neuropsychology*, 40(3), pp. 138–54.

4 Sun, W., Li, S., Jiang, Y., et al. (2018), 'A community-based study of sleep and cognitive development in infants and toddlers', *Journal of Clinical Sleep Medicine*, 14(6).

5 Nakagawa, M., Ohta, H., Shimabukuro, R., et al. (2021), 'Daytime nap and nighttime breastfeeding are associated with toddlers' nighttime sleep', *Scientific Reports*, 11, p. 3028.

6 Ibid.

7 LeBourgeois M. (2013), 'Circadian phase and its relationship to nighttime sleep in toddlers', *Journal of Biological Rhythms*, 28(5), pp. 322–31.

8 Etchell, A., Adhikari, A, Weinberg, L., et al. (2018), 'A systematic literature review of sex differences in childhood language and brain development', *Neuropsychologia,* 114, pp. 19–31.

Chapter 9

1 Huttenlocher, P. and Dabholkar, A. (1997), 'Regional differences in synaptogenesis in human cerebral cortex', *Journal of Comparative Neurology*, 387(2), pp. 167–78.

2 Luby, J., Barch, D., Belden, A., et al. (2012), 'Maternal support in early childhood predicts larger hippocampal volumes at school age', *Proceedings of the National Academy of Sciences Early Edition*, 109(8), pp. 2854–9.

3 Coulthard, H. and Sealy, A. (2017), 'Play with your food! Sensory play is associated with tasting of fruits and vegetables in preschool children', *Appetite*, 113, pp. 84–90.

4 Fisher, J. and Birch, L. (1999), 'Restricting access to palatable foods affects children's behavioral response, food selection, and intake', *American Journal of Clinical Nutrition*, 69(6), pp. 1264–72.

5 Mindell, J., Sadeh, A., Kwon, R., et al. (2013), 'Cross-cultural differences in the sleep of preschool children', *Sleep Medicine*, 14(12), pp. 1283–9.

6 Lask, B. (1988), 'Novel and non-toxic treatment for night terrors', *BMJ*, 297(6648), p. 592.

7 Montgomery, P., Burton, J., Sewell, R., et al. (2014), 'Fatty acids and sleep in UK children: subjective and pilot objective sleep results from the DOLAB study – a randomized controlled trial', *Journal of Sleep Research*, 23(4), pp. 364–88.

8 Tomasello, M. (2018), 'How children come to understand false beliefs: a shared intentionality account', *Proceedings of the National Academy of Sciences*, 115(34), pp. 8491–8.

9 Mischel, W. and Ebbesen, E. (1970), 'Attention in delay of gratification', *Journal of Personality and Social Psychology,* 16(2), p. 329.

10 Halil, K. and Burak, A., (2020), 'The association between parents' problematic smartphone use and children's speech delay', *Psychiatry and Behavioral Sciences,* 10(3), pp.110–15.

11 Twenge, J., Campbell, W., (2018), Associations between screen time and lower psychological well-being among children and adolescents: evidence from a population-based study', *Preventive Medicine Reports, 12,* pp. 271–283.

12 Strick, E. and Schubert, R., (1989), *Der Spielzeugfreie Kindergarten, Aktion Jugendschutz.*

Chapter 10

1 Nelson, C. A. and Jeste, S., 'Neurobiological perspectives on developmental psychopathology'. In: Rutter, M., Bishop, D., Pine, D., Scott, S., Stevenson, J., Taylor, E., et al. (eds) (2008), *Textbook on Child and Adolescent Psychiatry,* 5th edn, Blackwell Publishing: London.

2 Avants, B., Betancourt, L., Giannetta, J., et al. (2012), 'Early childhood home environment predicts frontal and temporal cortical thickness in the young adult brain', *Neuroscience 2012 Presentation,* programme: 908.02; poster: BBB25.

3 Huttenlocher, P. and Dabholkar, A. (1997), 'Regional differences in synaptogenesis in human cerebral cortex', *Journal of Comparative Neurology,* 387(2), pp. 167–78.

4 Mascola, A., Bryson, S. and Agras, W. (2010), 'Picky eating during childhood: a longitudinal study to age 11 years', *Eating Behaviour,* 11(4), pp. 253–7.

5 Ehrenberg, S., Leone, L., Sharpe, B., et al. (2019), 'Using repeated exposure through hands-on cooking to increase children's preferences for fruits and vegetables', *Appetite,* 142, p. 104347.

6 Flanders, J., Leo, V., Paquette, D., et al. (2009), 'Rough-and-tumble play and the regulation of aggression: an observational study of father–child play dyads', *Aggressive Behavior,* 35(4), pp. 285–95.

Index